Medicine & The Information Age

by Jeffrey S. Rose, MD

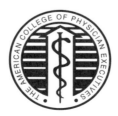

American College of Physician Executives
Tampa, FL

ISBN: 0-924674-57-1
Library of Congress Card Number: 97-77013

Printed in the United States of America by
Hillsboro Printing, Tampa, Florida

TABLE OF CONTENTS

This book introduces fundamental concepts of information systems and emphasizes skills, techniques, and abstractions for creating them and for managing resistance to them. It is a bit unconventional, as management books go, because it is not intended to "zap" you, "blockbust" you, hurtle you from one curve to another, shock you into a "paradigm shift," or teach you to swim with sharks. Rather, it's meant to ground you just long enough to give you a foundation knowledge of clinical information systems and to convince you of the critical importance of such systems to the survival and recovery of medical care in America.

It has been written for health care managers and educators, consultants, insurance executives, health plan/hospital chief information officers (CIOs), and clinical professionals, all of whom are considering new styles of care delivery and being irrevocably propelled into the world of computing. It has been purposefully aimed at fundamentals, because the sense I get from interactions with health industry leaders and practicing clinicians on the topic of information systems is that, while the benefits provided by technical books on the proper running of today's medical-information-business marathon are desired, many are uncomfortable asking someone to step into their office and show them something as basic as how to tie their new running shoes. Whether you work with patients, doctors, or information system developers, the concepts presented here will treat the queasiness felt when you see book titles such as *Business Wisdom of the Electronic Elite,*[1] *The Digital Economy,*[2] *Medical Nemesis,*[3] *Medicine on Trial,*[4] *Confessions of a Medical Heretic,*[5] and *Cybermedicine.*[6]

> *It has been written for health care managers and educators, consultants, insurance executives, health plan/hospital chief information officers (CIOs), and clinical professionals, all of whom are considering new styles of care delivery and being irrevocably propelled into the world of computing.*

Executives, managers, system developers, and analysts may wonder what a doctor has to offer on the topics of change and information systems. (They may even view doctors as impediments to the advancement of information technology; parts of the problem rather than the solution.*) Clinicians may be relieved to discover an empathic colleague writing in this area, but they may question whether anyone can bring healing, computers, and business together in a productive manner. My hope is that this curiosity will encourage you to read on.

---

*This is an unexpressed view, no doubt, seeing as we all get sick from time to time and, well, one never knows when one will want to be "liked" by the surgeon.

I must admit that I had clinical, administrative, and management experience when I began my work with information systems, but I was quite unfamiliar with computer jargon and large technical project processes. I was very comfortable with "liberal arts," intuition, interpretation, and medical history, but I had avoided computers, databases, statistics, and engineering.

I had the uneasy feeling, however, that the technology train was going to pull out of the station whether I was on it or not and that the information age would mean that clinicians and managers at all levels were going to need to "rethink" their structure and behavior in light of the new technology. (The astonishing success of many enlightened companies today is due to the use of innovative information technology as a vehicle for rethinking—not just reengineering—corporate work style, structure, and culture.)

I found that computer scientists had only slightly less empathy for clinicians' fears of information technology than did the clinicians for the computer scientists' concerns about surgical mishaps. Health care administrators were somewhere in between, intimidated by both "factions" and unsure how information technology could ever be properly used to benefit care providers and patients without "breaking the bank."

It seemed to me that traditional management methods were dying and being replaced by new information-enabled leadership and vision. I was relatively sure that old-style management, and old style medical practice, would not quietly fade into extinction and that, despite considerable rage, sobbing, screaming, and gnashing of teeth, those who thought through their *structure* and *culture* in light of information system capabilities and who retooled accordingly would prevail.

As I immersed myself in the concepts and language of information systems, I found that computer scientists had only slightly less empathy for clinicians' fears of information technology than did the clinicians for the computer scientists' concerns about surgical mishaps. Health care administrators were somewhere in between, intimidated by both "factions" and unsure how information technology could ever be properly used to benefit care providers and patients without "breaking the bank."

As the information-driven transformation of healing and of the health care industry occurs, the language and traditions of business, medicine, and computing must come together. A conceptual model that all three cultures can share for gaining a mutual understanding of one another's approaches, methods, and ideologies seems a prerequisite to cooperation and progress. I have attempted to establish "common ground" by presenting key elements of cross-cultural language and by comparing information system and management principles to *life processes*. (This may be the only "management" or "information systems" book in your library that is based on hundreds of millions of years of experience.) Knowledge of life processes and of the things that go wrong with them in humans is the basis of medicine; applicable in a broader sense to organization management are the magnificent ways in which equilibrium is maintained in the nonhuman living world.[7-9] Information is the core element of success in this equilibrium, just as it is in business and medicine.

References

1. James, G. *Business Wisdom of the Electronic Elite*. New York, N.Y.:Random House, 1996.
2. Tapscott, D. *The Digital Economy*. New York, N.Y.: McGraw-Hill, 1996.
3. Illich, I. *Medical Nemesis*. New York, N,Y.: Pantheon, 1976.
4. Inlander, C., and others. *Medicine on Trial: An Appalling Story of Ineptitude, Malfeasance, Neglect, and Arrogance*. New York, N.Y.: Prentice-Hall, 1988.
5. Mendelsohn, R. *Confessions of a Medical Heretic*. Chicago, Ill.: Contemporary Books, 1979.
6. Slack, W. *Cybermedicine: How Computing Empowers Doctors and Patients for Better Health Care*. San Francisco, Calif.: Jossey-Bass, 1997.
7. Starr, C., and Taggart, R. *Biology: The Unity and Diversity of Life, 6th Edition*. Belmont, California: Wadsworth Publishing Co., 1992.
8. Alberts, B., and others. *Molecular Biology of the Cell, Third Edition*. New York, N.Y.: Garland Publishers, Inc., 1994.
9. Attenborough, D. *Life on Earth, a Natural History*. Boston, Mass.: Little Brown and Co., 1979.

Chance, Necessity, Culture, and Change

If we want everything to remain as it is, it will be necessary for everything to change.—
Giuseppe Tomasi Di Lampedusa, Sicilian author, 1960.

Five decades have passed since the introduction of the first computer, Eniac 1, and the dawn of the information age. Automation and networks have dramatically altered everything in business from operations and planning to project execution and quality assurance, and have enabled the frenetic activities of a "reengineering revolution."[1,2] Developing information currency and leading the humans who save and spend it is defining new corporate champions and enabling cooperation and autonomy enterprise drivers in place of increasingly outmoded methods of control, authority, and competition.[3]

In the United States, medicine has become as much about business as about caring,[4] and, as unsettling as this may be, it is clear that financial viability and high performance in care delivery depend on successful collection and analysis of information. The medical marketplace is pressuring health care as a system to incorporate information technology into its processes in order to demonstrate clinical value and improved care outcomes. This is apparent from evaluation standards such as the National Committee for Quality Assurance's Health Plan Employer Data and Information Set (HEDIS) and "report cards" for health plans and insurance companies.[5-7] It is evident from insistence by health care payers on certification guidelines for remuneration and policies of determining clinician panel membership on the basis of individual resource utilization records. (As financiers of care are measured and scrutinized, so must be the providers of care themselves.) A stunning number of computerized medical record applications are being displayed at medical informatics conferences across the country, and the relatively new, but very robust "specialty" of medical informatics is reaching maturity.[8]

> *The medical marketplace is pressuring health care as a system to incorporate information technology into its processes in order to demonstrate clinical value and improved care outcomes.*

In these times of company mergers, hospital buy-outs, IPAs, PPOs, HMOs, managed care consortia, and community health affiliations, most organizations have found that simply joining forces or signing contracts is insufficient for meeting business goals and that the lack of integrated clinical information systems is a significant impediment to improving the quality and cost effectiveness of the medical care they seek to deliver. They are therefore designing or acquiring systems to enable greater efficiency, debating the merits and "return on investment" around dissemination of computers to examination rooms and physician offices, and deciding how to best leverage data they have already collected. They have realized that networked computing, if used by providers, facilitates coordination, cooperation, integration, and improvements in the quality of medical interactions and are hoping to use these same systems to provide better service, create customer loyalty, improve operational responsiveness, and enhance clinical effectiveness.[9-15] Because these goals depend on live "clinical systems in the care environment and not simple reporting databases or distant financial systems, clinical professionals are being propelled into new styles and organizations of care delivery, and irrevocably into the world of computing (and so are the patients who seek medical care.)

The only discernible end state of the information-driven cultural upheaval in medicine and business appears to be constant change. Indeed, the mind-boggling rate of technology evolution (somewhere near 10 million times the rate of biologic evolution) leads some to wonder if "perhaps we are careening into the future in a bobsled with no controls."[16] Clinicians can no longer keep up with the complexities of patient management and the explosion of new (and often ineffective) medical techniques, and health care administrators are no longer dealing with "static" organization components that could formerly be handled like ice cubes—frozen, collected, counted, rearranged, stuck together, and occasionally crushed. Today, everyone seems to be working with water; soon it will be vapor. Compared to the millennia-old practice of medicine, these changes are very sudden.

In these times of company mergers, hospital buy-outs, IPAs, PPOs, HMOs, managed care consortia, and community health affiliations, most organizations have found that simply joining forces or signing contracts is insufficient for meeting business goals and that the lack of integrated clinical information systems is a significant impediment to improving the quality and cost effectiveness of the medical care they seek to deliver.

The key impacts of information on organizations revolve around the enhanced ability to communicate knowledge in such a way that decision making can be decentralized, operational controls relaxed, accountability dispersed, and connections between previously separate activity centers established. The new information systems challenge traditional ideas about enterprise roles and structure, from the organization chart to bricks and mortar. In medicine, they facilitate a very fundamental change in the nature of the doctor/patient relationship, shifting it from one of professional beneficence, in which the patient surrenders control of health matters entirely to the "care" provider, to one of shared decision making between physician and patient based on high-quality "evidence" for treatment choices.

The practice of medicine is inherently information-intensive, and the potential for information systems to improve care delivery and enterprise functioning is alluring; the expense of networks and computing, however, make decisions in this regard financially treacherous. Smart acquisitions of information technology depend on the ability of clinical and administrative teams to understand their present operational formats and to achieve cooperative new configurations in the "digital" world.

Chance

Many successful companies in the current industrial climate seem to have a natural aptitude for using information systems to enable flexibility, individual responsibility, relatively unsupervised accountability, and an affinity for rapid change. The unique characteristics that have encouraged this behavior arose by chance and were "born" into environments that were hostile to it for many years; individuals with unconventional perspectives were outcasts, disharmonious with traditional control-and-command corporations. As these individuals found each other, however, they "grew up" and formed businesses based on their unique constructs, values, principles, attitudes, and technologic tools. This was analogous to the evolutionary impact of chance mutations in a gene pool, situating an altered organism for survival or extinction depending on surrounding environmental conditions.[17]

In health care, some clinicians foresaw the time when traditional approaches to medicine would not be viable, and early mutants in this area began unusual, even "heretical," practices, such as prepaid care, community rating for indemnity insurance, measurements of amount and utility of treatments, rewards for managing cost and quality instead of the number of procedures done or patients seen, shifts of care to teams, and focus on health promotion in addition to disease treatment.[18] This shift also created outcasts, similar to those who challenged old style corporate behavior, and brought new values and unique tools to the modern era.[19] The outcasts gradually found themselves thriving, and the results of their activities were actually altering the business environment for everyone in a fashion that only further favored their approach.

The practice of medicine is inherently information-intensive, and the potential for information systems to improve care delivery and enterprise functioning is alluring; the expense of networks and computing, however, make decisions in this regard financially treacherous.

Having "mutated," they were favored by a shifting environment; the mutation happened first and the advantage followed.

Recognition of the importance and advantage of these "mutant" qualities has not been lost on traditional medical enterprises, but they have faced the same problems other mature businesses encountered in revising norms to meet new challenges. Adapting to new external circumstances as an established and previously successful traditional "adult," with the same old genes, is hard to accomplish in a short time, but information system tools exist that can promote changes in the imprinted behavior patterns in health care more rapidly than ever before.

Necessity

Health care in America (and elsewhere) suffers terribly from problems in collecting, documenting, and analyzing clinical information and secondarily from the ravages of wasteful applications of technology and treatment when there is little sound basis for them.[20] The decisions each clinician makes hundreds of times each day are weakened further by the absence of well-organized, accessible, complete medical records at the moment the decisions are made.

Information technology is critical to alleviating at least three core health care system problems:

- Inadequate patient information in making clinical decisions.

- Inadequate evidence to guide diagnostic and treatment choices and to maximize effectiveness and value.

- Data toxicity: an overload of redundant, inaccurate, uninformative, or confusing "facts," leading to incorrect conclusions.

Social and economic pressures make it clear that it is the responsibility of clinicians, managers, and consumers to apply appropriate tools to the solution of these problems, well and immediately.

Culture and Change

The road to information competency and the "knowledge-based enterprise", however desirable, is littered with the carcasses of what should have been successful efforts and paved with well earned disasters.[21-25] (Carcasses and disasters are referred to as "experience.") Why is the process of implementing new information systems in many enterprises, and especially in health care, so often one of gore and mayhem?

There are two fundamental barriers to reaping the benefits of widespread information system use in health care. Both have already been witnessed in nonclinical enterprises, and both have much more to do with people than technology.

First, it is difficult to fuse modern information technology culture with traditional business culture, let alone archetypal medical culture. In the past, it was acceptable to keep the information "hackers" isolated in their cubicles, responding to random assignments and inquiries; generating claims, referrals, and professional resource utilization reports; and handling technology misadventures while executives managed "the business" and doctors treated patients.

Health care in America (and elsewhere) suffers terribly from problems in collecting, documenting, and analyzing clinical information and secondarily from the ravages of wasteful applications of technology and treatment when there is little sound basis for them.

Now, however, it is very apparent that clinicians and managers must become hackers to some extent and that the "techies" must in turn be helped to understand the business and processes of care. Most health care administrators have become painfully aware of this, and many clinical practitioners (who really do "manage" their businesses by virtue of the decisions they make on a moment-to-moment basis) have had to acknowledge a powerful but unfamiliar new clinical tool, the computer, in their midst.

Achieving this cross-cultural understanding and cooperation is not easy, because the methods and behavior of the management, clinical, and information technology communities are exercised using different languages and are based on different values.[26] The terminology integral to the information era has developed so swiftly that many established and very competent doctors and managers find themselves "out of touch." Suddenly "board room" is passé and "motherboard" is de rigueur. "Dictation" has given way to "speech recognition." The practice of voice-mailing oneself a reminder is "recursion." The "chart" is an "electronic health record," and clinical practice requires a modem as well as a stethoscope. Today's manager is signing "PCRs," requesting "ISDNs," looking at "prototypes," and pondering the mysteries of "LANs," and clinicians are using "results look-up" on the Internet, ordering "on-line," and communicating via e-mail.

First, it is difficult to fuse modern information technology culture with traditional business culture, let alone archetypal medical culture.

Caught in an expanding language gap, what manager hasn't experienced "mego" (my eyes glaze over) during an important technology team meeting, only to witness its damaging effect on morale? What clinician hasn't gotten edgy as training for use of a new office or hospital computer system approached (or didn't approach)?

This new technology enables a break from traditional management methods and familiar medical practice routines, and, at the same time, accentuates the need to communicate and to think in new ways. As Geoffrey James points out, "New leaders don't sound like typical dyed-in-the-wool suit executives. They use different words, draw different parallels, apply different imagery."[3] I would add that new clinicians don't sound like old doctors; they use new words, apply different principles, and communicate with their patients in different ways. In fact, I believe that they actually "think" differently.

If cross-cultural understanding and communication are lacking, it is nearly impossible for one group (information services) to produce something that pleases another group (clinical care providers) while at the same time meeting enterprise goals (management targets), regardless of how well intentioned all the participants are.

If cross-cultural understanding and communication are lacking, it is nearly impossible for one group (information services) to produce something that pleases another group (clinical care providers) while at the same time meeting enterprise goals (management targets), regardless of how well intentioned all the participants are.

The second difficulty lies in the fact that the product of the new technology, information, exceeds the willingness and ability of workers to cope with the real and perceived consequences of what can be discovered and evaluated. The use of computers and networks for collecting, analyzing, and sharing information can have significant detrimental social ramifications. Contrary to the expectation of improved human interaction and enhanced business performance, such systems can have an effect similar to the sudden merging of different countries; borders between co-existing business subcultures vanish, "currencies" mix and become confused, language differences introduce misunderstanding, philosophical and practical methods clash, and fears of domination and control arise.[24]

The term "subculture" is used here as a label for a collection of human behaviors in department, division, or functional areas that are linked by common tools, language, and abstract thought. The degree to which subculture mixing hinders enterprise function and growth depends on the amount of diversity at the time of intermingling, the willingness of occupational communities to trust or compromise, the ability of leaders to instill a common sense of purpose, and the desire to cooperate among previously segregated groups. The more autonomous, authoritative, independent, or powerful individuals are in a particular culture, the more threatened they may be by change and new information age processes. It is therefore little wonder that the application of information systems to centuries old traditions of medical practice has lagged behind its introduction in other industries. The rate-limiting step in the entire transition process is still human; confidence, power, security, autonomy, and equanimity are all threatened by what can now be discovered and communicated.

The second difficulty lies in the fact that the product of the new technology, information, exceeds the willingness and ability of workers to cope with the real and perceived consequences of what can be discovered and evaluated.

Whereas groups, divisions, departments, and individuals (including executives and neurosurgeons) could previously collect and sometimes hoard their information valuables, thereby maintaining a sense of importance, it is now apparent that this form of job security can't be guaranteed. "Fancy machinery" and "esoteric technology" are now manifesting themselves in ways that present enormous challenges to leaders, whose paramount duty is still to engage individuals and occupational communities in ways that promote trust and enhance performance, and to clinicians, whose job it is to provide compassionate, knowledgeable care for their patients.

Most managers and clinicians have developed skills for working with people in a relatively stable traditional environment, but advances in information system capabilities have intensified the emotional components of work, accelerated shifts in "power," and necessitated radical alterations in the ways in which many individuals accomplish tasks. Patients have more interest in and knowledge about their illnesses, doctors are shifting emphasis from "care" to prevention, and everyone is more than a little unsettled.

Information systems comprise one "major component" and four "minor components"; the major component is the collection of humans who use the minor components to accomplish their work.

Can the difficulties organizations have with information system-induced subculture mixing be understood in a more personal way with respect to medical culture? Are there accessible, straightforward reasons for the resistance to computers and software-based decision support in medical practice that could be comprehended and subsequently tackled in a direct manner? If so, how does one begin?

I believe the answer to both of these questions is yes, and this book provides the understanding and the tools to allow a good beginning.

Goal 1

The first and primary goal of this book is to help close the language gap. The unifying focus is core terminology, because without a solid base one cannot understand, let alone feel comfortable with, the complementary subcultures of an increasingly technical world. The book is intended to provide the germinal conceptual base needed to intelligently communicate with information systems professionals and to be at ease in asking for help.

...the most common reason for failure of information systems, regardless of professional domain, has everything to do with human behavior and little to do with anything else.

Managers and health professionals need not know all the new language to understand and relate more precisely, nor do they need exhaustive minutiae. This is why computer books, project development texts, and dictionaries can be unappealing. On the other hand, doctors and managers generally don't want bookshelves lined with guides for "dummies" and instructions for "idiots." However aptly titled, these texts may still go into greater detail than required. What I believe is needed, and hope to provide here, is a dignified, concise source of practical material that can be absorbed in pieces, between patients or meetings, and that is memorable without memorization.

Goal 2

The second goal of this work is to review the human factors and barriers involved in the use of information technology in business and medicine, focusing first on the key differences between management and technology subcultures and next on the effects of "information" on users. As changes in the "business" of health care occur, it becomes increasingly important for clinical teams to understand their structure and the principles of cooperation and change. Conceptualizing organizational structure and enterprise change processes in a way that fits more naturally into the information age allows one to deal in a more visionary and effective way with business operations and relationships.

There are numerous academic (ponderous) treatises on organizational factors influencing the introduction of technology, with attention to psychology, sociology, psychosociology, social anthropology, organizational behavior, organizational management, and cognitive science. These treatises contain mind-boggling considerations of vertical versus horizontal communication pathways and processes with models of change such as "research, development, and diffusion," "problem solving," and "social interaction" and names like "Kolb-Frohman Model" and "Roger's Classic Diffusion Theory." Some are comprehensive and excellent.[21,26,27] Many are impractical and unreadable. In several instances, these articles and books appear to have been written by academicians who profess solutions to problems they have sought to escape by going into academia or who want to "lecture on navigation while the ship is going down."[28] This book is intended to be a sensible guide, with material that is easy to understand and recall; although professorial works are referenced from time to time, their complexities are not dwelled upon.

Going Deep

Because the major goal of this book is to help individuals in medical, business, and information technology cultures understand one another's language and thought processes, I have frequently relied on metaphors and analogies to communicate. I believe these enhance appreciation for other perspectives, because knowing something "metaphorically" confers an intuitive understanding with levels of meaning most harmonious with the reader's own insights and experiences. Clinicians and individuals in leadership positions seem to have a natural aptitude for comprehending new ideas and absorbing knowledge presented in this way.

The Tenth Century contemplative Muslim philosophical and literary movement called Sufism used very powerful "teaching stories" to impart knowledge. The story of the Water Melon Hunter is a perfect way to introduce this work:

A man wandered from his own country into a world known as the Land of the Fools. He observed denizens of the foreign world running terrified from a field where they were reaping wheat. The frightened individuals proclaimed that there was a "monster" in the field.

The man looked at the monster and observed a watermelon. He "killed" the monster; cutting the watermelon from its stem and slicing it into pieces, which he then began to eat.

The "Fools" became even more frightened of the man than they had been of the monster, fearing he would kill them next, and they banded together and drove him away with pitchforks.

At another time, another man similarly strayed into the Land of the Fools and observed the same situation. Instead of killing the monster, however, he shared the Fool's fear, agreeing that the melon must be dangerous, and, by retreating with them, he gained their confidence. He spent a long time with them in their houses, until, little by little, he could teach them the basic facts that would enable them not only to lose their fear of melons, but even to cultivate them themselves.[29]

Both of the men knew the facts. They understood what the melon was, how it consisted of rind and sweet fruit and productive seeds, and that it was not dangerous. Only the wiser man realized that facts alone were insufficient to impart knowledge to a fearful people. The same is true of the facts and fears that surround the introduction and acceptance of new information system technology into established environments.

Handling the Book

Information systems comprise one "major component" and four "minor components"; the major component is the collection of humans who use the minor components to accomplish their work.

Part I: The first section of this book is intended to "set the stage"—to illuminate the change required in medicine and to convince health care professionals that they can and must participate. It examines what is happening in modern healing and why, and proposes what is needed to make things better.

It takes the form of a case presentation, similar to what might be composed by a compulsive intern for reporting to the attending physician on hospital rounds, and deals extensively with the role information systems can play in healing a very sick patient, Dr. Iatros, (iatros is the Greek term for physician). Every attempt has been made to keep this presentation authentic, while at the same time accessible and enjoyable for nonclinical readers. The cultural barriers to use of information systems in medicine are dealt with, and recommendations for healing health care using such systems prescribed. (The remainder of the book is intended to impart language and instill new concepts to make the necessary changes in your setting.)

Part II: This section concentrates on providing select "facts" about the "minor components" to confer an understanding of "hardware" (computers and other physical devices), "software" (instructions that tell hardware what to do), "networks" (wires or other communication media linking hardware), and "information" (data one puts in, takes out, evaluates, or sends around). The intent of these chapters is to provide an understanding of information systems that is on par with the understanding of the melon by the man in the Sufi story and to act as a primer for the lexicon that constitutes the final section of the book.

Part III: This section tackles the "major component"—people. Its focus is on universal human characteristics and on the delicate management of the challenges presented by information riches. It addresses the great importance of culture, emotion, enterprise structure, and organizational change as they relate to information technology. Although its emphasis is less on medical culture and more on business and information technology culture, it is very important, because the most common reason for failure of information systems, regardless of professional domain, has everything to do with human behavior and little to do with anything else. Understanding the melon is necessary but insufficient for dealing with the fears of those who lack the same understanding.

Part IV: These chapters pull knowledge from earlier sections together in a practical review of the language and the processes of information system projects. They provide insights into more concrete aspects of project planning, management, and implementation. (Clinicians may find this of less interest, but it will be useful if one participates in the design of an information system or wishes to better understand the trials and tribulations of colleagues who are trying to make development and implementation of new technology look easy.) Newcomers to the processes of system development may find this section essential, and those more seasoned in this regard may find the tribulations detailed here familiar and rather amusing.

Lexicon: This is the core reference section of the book, a "super" dictionary of fundamental terminology to establish one's information system verbal persona. The nuances included in this lexicon serve to make the language more meaningful, conferring more than just a jargon veneer. I have repeatedly observed that comprehending these terms and their delicate hidden meanings confers on leaders a Zen-like ability to cope with the trials and tribulations of project and company management and entices generally serious clinicians with humor that is essential in times of difficult change.

Anything Else?

This book will also amuse those in a wider reading audience who, regardless of profession, enjoy the peculiarities of language. (If you are curious about the concept of a "reading audience," you are in this group.)

Science and technology multiply around us. To an increasing extent they dictate the languages in which we speak and think. Either we use those languages, or we remain mute.—J.G. Ballard, English novelist, 1974.

References

1.   Hammer, M., and Stanton, S. *The Reengineering Revolution: A Handbook.* New York, N.Y.: Harper Collins, 1995.
2.   Martin, J. *An Information System Manifesto.* Upper Saddle River, N.J.: Prentice-Hall, 1984.
3.   James, G. *Business Wisdom of the Electronic Elite.* New York, N.Y.: Random House, 1996.
4.   Halvorson, G. *Strong Medicine.* New York, N.Y.: Random House, 1993.

5. "How Good Is Your Health Plan." *Consumer Reports*, Aug. 1996, pp. 25-42.

6. "Are HMOs the Right Prescription?" *U.S. News and World Report*, Oct. 13, 1977, pp. 60-78.

7. "Does Your HMO Stack Up?" *Newsweek*, June 24, 1996, pp. 56-62.

8. Van Bemmel, J., and Musen, M. *Handbook of Medical Informatics*. Bohn, Germany: Springer-Verlag, 1997.

9. Tierney, W., and others. "The Effect on Test Ordering of Informing Physicians of the Charges for Outpatient Diagnostic Tests." *New England Journal of Medicine* 322(21):1524-5, May 24, 1990.

10. Tierney, W., and others. "Computer Predictions of Abnormal Test Results: Effects on Outpatient Testing." *JAMA* 259(8):1194-8, Feb. 26, 1988.

11. Tierney, W., and others. "Physician Inpatient Order Writing on Microcomputer Workstations: Effects on Resource Utilization." *JAMA* 269(3):379-83, Jan. 20, 1993.

12. Shea, S., and others. "Computer General Informational Messages Directed to Physicians: Effect on Length of Hospital Stay." *JAMIA* 2(1):58-64, Jan.-Feb. 1995.

13. Brownbridge, G., and others. "Patient Reactions to Doctors'Computer Use in General Practice Consultations." *Social Science and Medicine* 20(1):47-52, 1985.

14. McDonald, C. "The Barriers to Electronic Medical Record Systems and How to Overcome Them." *JAMIA* 4(3):213-221, May-June 1997.

15. Schriger, D., and others. "Implementation of Clinical Guidelines Using a Computer Charting System." *JAMA* 278(19):1985-9, Nov. 19, 1997.

16. Arthur, W. "How Fast Is Technology Evolving?" *Scientific American* 276(2):105, Feb. 1997.

17. Monod, J. *Chance and Necessity: An Essay on the Natural Philosophy of Modern Biology*. New York, N.Y.: Knopf, 1971.

18. Smillie, J. Can Physicians Manage Quality and Costs of Health Care? *The Story of the Permanente Medical Group*. New York, N.Y.: McGraw-Hill, 1991

19. Starr, P. *The Social Transformation of American Medicine*. New York, N.Y.: Harper Collins Publishers, 1982.

20. Eddy, D., and Billings, S. "The Quality of Medical Evidence: Implications for Quality of Care." *Health Affairs* 7(1):19-32, Spring 1988

21. Lorenzi, N., and others. "Antecedents of the People and Organizational Aspects of Medical Informatics: Review of the Literature." *JAMIA* 4(2):79-93, March-April 1997.

22. Williams, S. "Microchips Versus Stethoscopes: Calgary Hospital MDs Face Off Over Controversial Computer System." *Canadian Medical Association Journal* 147(10):1534-40,43-4,47, Nov. 15, 1992.

23. News, D. "London Perspective: Unhealthy Computer Systems." *Lancet* 341(8855):1269-70, May 15, 1993.

24. Rotmon, B., and others. "A Randomized Controlled Trial of a Computer-Based Physician Workstation in an Outpatient Setting: Implementation Barriers to Outcome Evaluation." *JAMIA* 3(5):340-8, Sept.-Oct. 1996.

25. Liebowitz, J., Editor *Journal of Failure and Lessons Learned in Information Technology Management*, New York, N.Y.:Cognizant Communication Corp.

26. Schein, E. *Organizational Culture and Leadership*, Second Edition. San Francisco, Calif.: Jossey-Bass Publishers, 1992.
27. Lorenzi, N. *Organizational Aspects of Health Informatics: Managing Technological Change.* New York, N.Y.: Springer-Verlag, 1995.
28. Boren, J. in Jarmin, C., *The Guinness Book of Poisonous Quotes.* Chicago, Ill.: Contemporary Books, 1993, p. 214
29. Shah, I. *The Way of the Sufi.* London, England: Penguin Books, Ltd., 1968, p. 227.

Acknowledgments

Recognizing those who have helped one attain the experience and the knowledge that form the foundation of a book is perhaps the most pleasurable element of authorship. It is also a bit treacherous because of the potential for inadvertent exclusion. I considered deviating from convention with some specific "disknowledgments," inscribing those who made professional growth exceptionally difficult, reasoning that with this approach anyone who was excluded would feel lucky rather than unappreciated. I ultimately decided that such an alternative was rather unkind, in addition to being too lengthy, and so I proceed with some specific thanks and the hope that all readers acquainted with me will assume that I am thankful to them as well, listed or not.

The executive management ability and vision in the Rocky Mountain Division of Kaiser Permanente are unique in my experience, and I am grateful to Toby Cole, Andy Wiesenthal, Kate Paul, Mike Alexander, John Pappas, and Bill Marsh for supporting me in the position of leadership from which stem many of the observations presented in this work. I extend special thanks to the outstanding members of the development and implementation teams of our clinical information system, in particular Pat Bow, Jo Comstock, Steven Kay, Ben Chao, Gary Brown, Kerry Davidson, Brian Randall, Janie Poteet, Chuck Roberts, Gregg Hushka, and Casey Webster. I deeply appreciate the work of John Fedack, Aaron Snyder, Dave Thomas, and Ted Palen, each notable for distinguished patience, alarming persistence, and absolving good humor.

I am very grateful for the efforts of all of my fellow clinicians in Colorado Kaiser Permanente, more than 250 of whom thought through our system with the team and gave considerable personal time to the project. I particularly appreciate the efforts of our germinal "resource committee," the follow-on "core committee," and the extra work of Doug Warriner, Elsa Swyers, Jack Scholz, Peter Dwork, Cheryl Rogers, Mike Chase, and Andy Lum. I salute the revered clinicians who continue to help us through the tribulations of early application delivery and revision, in particular the pioneers at our East Medical Facility. Thanks as well to the system analysts, designers, developers, functional area owners, testers, trainers, and technical writers who labored in the effort. Special thanks to the entire T.J. Watson research team in New York, which applied considerable ingenious talent to meeting clinical needs with information technology, especially Ifay Chang, Houtan Aghili, Rich Mushlin, Eric Mays, Kevin MacAuliffe, Art Amman, Guy Hochgesang, and Rose Williams.

I particularly appreciate my friend John Dewey and his consistently visionary views on information systems in health care. I am thankful as well for the support of colleagues George Peredy, Ted Cooper, Simon Cohn, Homer Chin, Steve Miller, Allan Khoury, Glenn Rennels, and Lance Lang, and for the patient teaching of my technical friends, Abdul Malik Shakir, Steven Gee, Jansin Lee, Bob Haas, Dave Minch, and Randi Ferraro. My deep thanks and admiration go to Ron Williams, who is spectacular proof that superb technologists can be among the most spiritual and humane of our species.

I am enormously indebted to John Wolfe, who shepherded things along and offered sage advice over the years; to Jon Otsuki, who counselled behind the scenes; and to Wendy Rubel, who threw me in front of large audiences as a method of getting me to organize my experiences with large-scale system development in the health care arena.

I particularly appreciate the contributions of Marianne Gapinski, Cathy Anderson, and Bruce Fisch, who each carefully reviewed early manuscripts and made many helpful suggestions, and I am exceptionally grateful to my friend and colleague Kim Adcock, who helps me keep my focus on the crucial role of appropriate clinical decision making in high-quality health care. I am very thankful to Wes Curry at ACPE and to Karen Schaeffer for their editorial work, and to Andy Pasternack at Jossey-Bass for his enthusiastic support.

I think it is also appropriate to use this space to express my admiration for the efforts and teachings of the crusaders referenced in the following chapters who have sought to develop clinical computing and raise consciousness about evidence-based health care, in particular David Eddy, Donald Berwick, John Wennberg, George Halvorson, David Plotkin, Paul Clayton, Jim Cimino, Clement McDonald, Lawrence Weed, Christopher Chute, Kent Spackman, William Tierney, Mark Musen, and Mark Tuttle.

Most important, I am eternally grateful for the encouragement and sacrifices of Barbara, Colin, and Ellary, my extraordinary family, who allowed countless evening and weekend hours of isolation to write this book, shared the stresses and strains of large-scale project management that I thoughtfully brought home, and tolerated the absences required to obtain and refine my clinical system knowledge.

Information Systems and Medicine

Part 1

During medical school and training, doctors relate the results of patient evaluations to attending physicians in the form of case presentations. Since the introduction of problem-oriented charting in the early 1970s, these presentations have loosely the format here, wherein **subjective** information related by the patient (comprising complaints, history of the illness, allergies, medications, psychosocial conditions, family, health risk, and educational and developmental histories), **objective** information gathered by the clinician (comprising vital sign measurements and physical examination findings), **assessment** of the illness (comprising diagnosis and discussion of the rationale for the determination), and **plan** (containing orders for treatment and recommendations) are documented. (These notes are often called **soap** notes by clinicians.)

The patient in this case (Dr. Iatros) represents an amalgam of American medical practitioners, ranging from traditional fee-for-service providers to clinicians in staff-model health maintenance organizations. Most of the symptoms and findings are applicable to all of the styles and methods of practice. Similarly, the insights and judgments considered

We must bear in mind that medicine is not a natural science, either pure or applied. The methods of science are used all the time in combating disease, but medicine itself belongs much more to the realm of social sciences, because the goal is social. Disease has influenced the course of history, economic, social, political; has devastated entire countries; has stopped wars, wiping out victor and victim. It presented a challenge to religion, science and philosophy, which were called upon to interpret disease, and to give men power over it.—Henry Sigerist, Medical Historian, 1951.

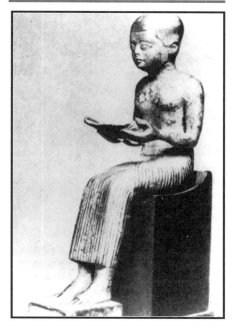

here represent a collection of evidence and evaluation by experts in medicine, epidemiology, medical economics, and medical history (their names and relevant works are noted at the conclusion of the case).

Language will be a major focus of the chapters that follow this case, and, in the interest of lexical clarity, I must point out that the term "managed care" is a popular misnomer that has been associated with maladaptive, poorly understood, shallow, financially driven efforts of cost control applied to health care. Truly "managed" care can only be delivered if appropriately educated individuals obtain and responsibly act on information. Controlling can be done with few data and less understanding; managing requires information in its complete form.

It's information, therefore, on which the future of health care is fundamentally dependent.

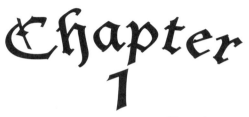

Chapter 1

The strange case of Dr. Iatros

---

*Mr. Spock : "Logic and practical information
do not seem to apply here."
Dr. McCoy: "You admit that?"
Mr. Spock: "To deny the facts would be illogical, Doctor."*

—*Star Trek*, "A Piece of the Action," 1968.

General Information

Dr. Iatros is a distinguished elderly patient of mixed ethnicity and strong Greek heritage who has been brought to the hospital by his brother, a health care administrator. The history of illness has been obtained primarily from the patient, who seems to be a credible historian (lucid, intelligent, articulate, and thoughtful), despite considerable nervousness during the interview. Some input was obtained from his brother (this latter source is noted when relevant).

Subjective Findings

Chief Complaints

The patient complains of weight loss, agitation, exhaustion, and feeling WADAO (weak and dizzy all over). He states, "I have no more energy. The world around me is spinning out of control, and I am broke and broken. I can't eat or sleep. No one understands me, treats me with the reverence I deserve, or cares about my dilemma."

"I have been playing as hard in this game as I possibly can, following the rules, but suddenly it seems as if I'm playing on a busy freeway instead of a field, and the game will be forfeited if I go out of bounds."

History of the Present Illness

The patient reports excellent health until approximately 1975, when recurrent symptoms of restlessness, fearfulness, insomnia, and excessive perspiration appeared. He concurrently experienced inability to concentrate, difficulty recalling facts needed to treat patients, and a pervasive sense of intellectual burden in his profession because of a plethora of new medications, unfamiliar diagnostic tests, and emerging therapeutic modalities.

He expresses anger over allegations by observers of health care, such as Ivan Illich, who asserted: "Medical bureaucracy creates ill health by increasing stress, by multiplying disabling dependence, by generating new painful needs, by lowering levels of tolerance for discomfort or pain, by reducing the leeway that people are wont to concede to an individual when he suffers, and by abolishing even the right to self-care."[1] He was also pained by comments such as those of family member Robert Mendelsohn, who asserted: "Modern medicine is now better geared for killing people than it is for healing them."[2]

Dr. Iatros associates most of the symptoms temporally with developing financial difficulties secondary to restriction of fees and denial of reimbursements by insurance companies and to the inability of his patients to pay for services out of pocket.

He had always been paid for performing procedures, seeing patients, ruling out diseases that might possibly be causing problems (regardless of likelihood), and generally "doing things"; he began to deeply resent restrictions on his methods imposed by "nonphysician purse-strings controllers"

He had always been paid for performing procedures, seeing patients, ruling out diseases that might possibly be causing problems (regardless of likelihood), and generally "doing things"; he began to deeply resent restrictions on his methods imposed by "nonphysician purse-strings controllers" (the brother rolled his eyes at this point in the interview). His attempts to balance finances without compromising what he believes to be "optimum quality" care raised ethical dilemmas for him, which added to his anxiety. He lost his appetite and has experienced a gradual weight loss over the past decade.

At around this time, utilization and case management staff, used predominantly by payers for care (mostly employers, insurance companies, and managed care programs) increasingly demanded proof of the clinical value of Dr. Iatros' costly services. (It made some sense to him that basing his compensation on the outcomes of services was reasonable, but he experienced great frustration trying to prove the merit of his actions because the results of his interventions were not precisely recorded or easily recoverable.) Because little reliable information about outcomes was available, those who paid his fees began to enforce arbitrary payment restrictions and to determine which doctors would be eligible to participate as providers in their plan based on their resource utilization records (test ordering and drug prescriptions). They intermittently denied payment on an unpredictable basis, assessing and weighting some costs inordinately while completely ignoring others. They also confused him with multiple restrictions on which drugs or treatments he could administer, depending on which plans he or his patients belonged to, such that he never really knew if he was complying or not. This practice ran counter to hundreds of years of tradition and incited some of the less ethical members of his profession to falsify data or to actually withhold proper treatment to look favorable in the numbers and to maintain profit. He experienced agitation and the gradual onset of insomnia.

Dr. Iatros notes that the outcry of the public about rising costs of care during this period and general dissatisfaction about the health care system resulted in the emergence of "managed care" (more aptly termed "managed costs"). Today, however, he notes that widespread dissatisfaction exists with the new paradigm, augmented by professional misery introduced with the controls.[3] He reports that he has occasionally wondered if patients really need all of his expensive ministrations. (His brother pointed out that nearly 50 percent of physicians surveyed by the American Medical Association in 1989 believed their patients were requesting unnecessary treatment.[4]) Legal, media, and public expectations seem to mandate perfect diagnostic accuracy and a full application of possible therapy (regardless of cost). Because so few data about efficacy are available for analysis and, when available, are highly biased because of their close association with reimbursement, he feels ignoring the issue is the best approach.

If he uses more efficient systems, orders fewer tests, performs fewer procedures, or encourages self-care through advice, which obviates the need for a patient visit, his reward is reduced income and patients who are confused and angry.

Despite his best efforts to contain costs it has become quite apparent that no company, group, individual, or society in general can afford him as he currently functions. If he uses more efficient systems, orders fewer tests, performs fewer procedures, or encourages self-care through advice, which obviates the need for a patient visit, his reward is reduced income and patients who are confused and angry. Working harder and longer has become increasingly stressful, bringing hours of financially and emotionally unrewarding efforts. In the past year, for the first time since 1985, his entire family experienced a diminution in income, some members by as much as 20 percent. Physicians in Dr. Iatros' family who had never been paragons of physical and emotional health, despite their calling, were seeking help for stress and applying for disability insurance benefits in record numbers.[2,5]

Dr. Iatros presented to the emergency department in 1991 and on several other occasions thereafter. Precipitating events for these urgent visits included: threats of massive health care reform; application of new rigid external criteria for reimbursement; mandates for duplicative, wasteful paperwork; press allegations of unethical behavior; and political recrimination for failure to attend to the health needs of significant portions of the population.

Legal, media, and public expectations seem to mandate perfect diagnostic accuracy and a full application of possible therapy (regardless of cost).

He was greatly disturbed at this time by the view of medical practice as a "business," as it had always seemed so much more sanctified than that; caring for patients had become serving "customers." The long-term patient loyalty that he had previously enjoyed was interrupted as his patients were shuffled between provider groups and employee health insurance plans as dictated by outside circumstances. He feels like a hostage, controlled by policies, mandates, and whims of enterprise "bean counters" who handle capital expenditures and don't interact with patients.

Dr. Iatros found it nearly impossible to please patients and meet their expectations while at the same time doing the right things for them and controlling costs. He is frustrated by the increasing number of patients who are seeking "alternative" medicine approaches and "natural" remedies that he sees as unscientific.

Dr. Iatros notes that public expectation clearly equates more tests, x-rays, medicines, and treatments with high quality of care; even when he knows the right thing to do (or not do) he cannot act, because he fears displeasing or alienating clients. On top of it all, his patients were also coming to him with expectations set by information and misinformation from newspapers, books, television and radio advertising, and from searches of the Internet, where "science and snake oil tend to look remarkably similar."[6] This is a very sensitive and stressful issue for him, because he interacts daily with individuals who think they are ill or are desirous of the best care as they see it, regardless of cost.[7] (Some of these same individuals are likely to opt to cancel their health insurance so they can afford a new car, buy cigarettes, or purchase a handgun.)

"Everyone still wants my very best, most technologically advanced services, but no one wants to pay for them," Dr. Iatros complains, "and, if I reasonably refuse to do something I feel is unnecessary and fail to satisfy patients, they either leave my practice or seek counsel to discredit me for denial of care or malpractice." Between patient demands and the fear of legal or financial reprisal, performance of every possible diagnostic test or application of every treatment on every patient seemed unavoidable.

The consistent assessments of Dr. Iatros from visit to visit in the emergency department were: anxiety over dealing with patient demands for expensive unnecessary diagnostic tests, pressure related to keeping up with medical knowledge, and the stress of survival in an environment with clearly diminishing resources. (Records of the visits are, of course, unavailable at this time, but the brother relates that one observer commented on the apparent difficulty Dr. Iatros had separating practices that were truly good for patients from those good for paying off a large mortgage; most opinions suggested this phenomenon was due to ignorance rather than greed.)

According to his brother, Dr. Iatros became extremely agitated when the alarm was sounded about the fact that per capita expenditures for health care in the United States were the highest of any country in the world and were rising at nearly twice the rate of inflation every year. He began raving about "decapitation" and claiming he was being savaged by charlatans and usurers and being unfairly treated by the media. Dr. Iatros' brother also said that, at about this time, the agitation was intensified by the observation that complete elimination of all of the external reasons Dr. Iatros had invoked to explain rising medical costs, including drug company profits, research expenses, administrative salaries, and support staff costs, would still fail to contain growing national expenditures for health care.[8] (Physician salaries, the brother related, could also be completely eliminated from the equation without significant gains in cost control; the direct costs of paying providers for their services accounted for only 15 percent of the total health care bill.)[9]

He was greatly disturbed at this time by the view of medical practice as a "business," as it had always seemed so much more sanctified than that; caring for patients had become serving "customers."

WADAO first appeared in 1978, when experts suggested that 80-90 percent of the health care decisions that Dr. Iatros made were ungrounded in any scientific evidence of effectiveness and were driving the enormous costs of the system. The experts observed that the vast majority of ill patients being seen would recover without any medical intervention whatsoever.[9-1] It appeared to be more than just Dr. Mendelsohn's opinion that "more than 90 percent of modern medicine could disappear from the face of the earth—doctors, hospitals, drugs, equipment—and the effect would be immediate and beneficial."[2]

One week prior to the current admission, the patient began to experience lapses of cognition and extreme difficulty making decisions about patients because of insufficient information. He became exceptionally worried that illnesses and even deaths might result from his lack of patient records and from his ignorance of which interventions posed more risk than benefit for his patients.

...complete elimination of all of the external reasons Dr. Iatros had invoked to explain rising medical costs, including drug company profits, research expenses, administrative salaries, and support staff costs, would still fail to contain growing national expenditures for health care.

Questioned about previous use of computers or information system technology, Dr. Iatros became agitated and flushed. He glanced warily at his brother and asserted that no computers he had ever seen were easy to use or worked for his purposes, although he often had clerks or nurses look things up for him.

He maintained there is no way he would ever type anything, because he never learned to type, was above typing, couldn't relate to patients in a compassionate way with a computer in the room because it would interfere with his warmth and patient bonding (patients wouldn't like it), and didn't have time anyway because he had to see patients so rapidly these days to keep solvent. (His brother noted that prior efforts on his part to present more complete patient hospital data via computer to Dr. Iatros were coolly rebuffed. On isolated occasions where computerized information was made available in the ambulatory setting, Dr. Iatros complained that there was "too much stuff to read it and the subtleties he liked to interject about nonmedical patient issues were missing.")

Past Medical History

Allergies and Adverse Reactions

- Agitation in reaction to direction by others, especially nonclinicians

- Hives and combative behavior as reaction to challenges to professional opinions.

- Shortness of breath in reaction to loss of income or threat of malpractice.

- Rash as reaction to "alternative" health approaches.

Medications

- Prozac® (for depression).

- Tagamet® (for peptic ulcers).

- Ritalin® (for alertness over long hours).

- Multiple anti-anxiety agents and sedatives (for nervousness and sleep).

(Patient has prescription bottles in paper bag; will retrieve dosage and strength later.)

Psychosocial Factors

- Moderate alcohol and cigarette use, unusually high rate of narcotic drug abuse compared to other professionals in the same socioeconomic class, higher than expected risk of suicide (twice the risk of nonphysician white Americans).[12,13]

- Ongoing grief reaction over loss of autonomy and death of traditional hospitals.

- Dysfunctional adjustment syndrome, with associated severe inflexibility characteristics (see family history).

- Past psychological testing shows extremely high motivation and intelligence, strong work ethic, tolerance for sleep deprivation, ability to endure professional humiliation for short periods, generally well-developed moral character, moderate perfectionism, extreme fear of failure, and inability to tolerate change. It also indicates advanced ability to make decisions without adequate information, but equally strong difficulties gaining "big picture perspective."

Health Risks

- Exposure to infectious disease and workplace hazards.

- Legislative accidents and stupidity (specifically, mandated treatments, hospital lengths of stay based on emotion— medicine as practiced by lawyers and politicians).

- Litigation trauma (unwarranted and warranted malpractice suits, with decisions based on emotion by a jury—medicine as practiced by the public).

Family History

(Only selected important elements of the family history bearing on Dr. Iatros' current condition are reviewed here. They are related because they illuminate certain behavior patterns, methods, and traits that point to substantial resistance to change, to adherence to old and ineffectual practices, and to a tradition of professional entitlement. They also suggest potential in the lineage for reason and innovation, which may affect prognosis.)

Ancestors

A heated debate was recorded between the God, Thoth, who delivered the writing capability to man, and the venerable older humans of the Egyptian civilization as to the effect this newfangled interface, writing, would have on thought, skills and nuances of story-telling, and the ritualistic handing down of verbal information as it had always been done before.

Dr. Iatros has a long and distinguished family history, dating back to the appearance of *Homo habilis*, possibly with roots in the late Paleolithic era, when humankind became users of crude instruments.[14] (Early use of axes and arrowheads unquestionably gave rise to trauma interventions.) Spiritual and religious healing were the norm among early family members, with occasional uprooting of demonstrably effective treatments (some herbs, fracture immobilization, removal of spears, and the like). Patients themselves often knew appropriate remedies to use, reserving trips to the doctor for advanced or dire illness or for application of curses to their enemies.

The importance of the physician, or shaman as he or she was called early on, had everything to do with magic, incantation, dance, and recompense for humans displeasing spirits or offending the gods. Patients of shaman seemed to get better or worse regardless of incantations, sometimes actually surviving direct interventions but always owing improvement to the doctor and decline to the degree of dissatisfaction on the part of the polytheistic powers of the culture. Charges were generally minimal. Home care was the rule, and, early on, the sickest patients were gathered into groups to die in primordial hospitals. (Dr. Iatros insightfully noted the persistence of this latter tradition in present times.)

Medical Records and Rationale

Human medical knowledge was orally passed among family members for many millennia, but everything changed with the invention of writing on paper. Egyptian relatives created paper from papyrus reeds along the Nile and used it for recording case histories. (A heated debate was recorded between the God, Thoth, who delivered the writing capability to man, and the venerable older humans of the Egyptian civilization as to the effect this newfangled interface, writing, would have on thought, skills and nuances of story-telling, and the ritualistic handing down of verbal information as it had always been done before.) After a few hundred years of trying, the writers won out, and the earliest clinical writing appears in the great medical papyri from about 1500 BC. (The lead portion of papyri was called the protokolon, origin of the word "protocol.")

Paper medical records were created about the time two-wheeled transportation was invented. Medical, surgical, and obstetric-gynecologic papyri, written in hieratic script, clearly demonstrate some rationality to medical practice and basic understanding and reliance on anatomic, physiologic, and medicinal elements of healing associated with clinical observation and deduction. They relay methods of treatment, including pharmacy, and give fascinating case records as examples of treatment regimens.[15] (They are also easier to decipher, despite the symbolic unfamiliarity of hieroglyphics, than most paper medical records today.) The argument over how to transmit and document medical history and knowledge in general represents primitive evidence in the family lineage of difficulty with change and especially with new technology.

> *The fundamental element, which cannot be overemphasized, was that doctors not only supported patients spiritually during the healing process, but also repeated and recorded basic practices that proved beneficial.*

The fundamental element, which cannot be overemphasized, was that doctors not only supported patients spiritually during the healing process, but also repeated and recorded basic practices that proved beneficial. The gods were still responsible for deaths, and physicians were deeply revered for their efforts and spiritual ties. Imhotep, for example, the physician to the pharaohs, was ultimately deified, becoming the minor god Ptah (pictured on the page that introduced Part I of this book), according to some historians. Doctor descendants found this quite reasonable and assumed follow-on entitlement to deification for all time, for all healers (see Hippocrates below.) In other words, they thought about what they were doing in a rational way. They had ample opportunity for such thinking during multiple wars, many dynasties, and an impressive number of plagues. Even doctors with miserable track records could earn a living by going into mummification, extracting viscera through incisions and brains through nostrils, thereby learning some anatomy. Their efforts contributed to the relating of anatomic structures to explanations of disease in a more empirical fashion, departing from the notion that all illness was due entirely to some god's anger.

The Egyptian family's Chinese brethren, meanwhile, were sticking sharp objects into patients to balance Yin and Yang, not surprisingly discovering the circulatory system in the process. (The Chinese family was also thought to have tried out the procedure known as inoculation, relevant later in this discussion, by blowing powdered pus from smallpox lesions up the nostrils of their most special patients as a preventive measure.) Considerable ongoing family discord over who figured out circulation, and what the pulse was, led to bickering between the Egyptian medical society and the Emperor Ti College of Physicians, carried on later by Drs. Galen, Celsius, and Hippocrates. The fighting and competing finally came to an end when English descendant William Harvey decided he discovered circulation 4,000 years later. This contentiousness is not to be overlooked when considering the current patient's condition.

Hippocrates and the Oath

A singularly important Hippocratic observation of great relevance to Dr. Iatros' current condition is, "Our natures are the physicians of our diseases," referring to the fact that patients seemed to progress naturally with their illnesses, regardless of physician interventions

Of prime importance in the patient's family tree, from the standpoint of the origin of his many present problems, is his most famous relative, Hippocrates of Greece. Most of the work and writing attributed to Hippocrates probably originated with his colleagues and friends and were enshrined in a set of principles and practices collectively referred to as the "Hippocratic tradition." (It is unlikely that his teachings spread widely during his lifetime or had great immediate impact, however, as Romans got along quite well for some 600 years without doctors, according to Pliny the Elder.[17])

Hippocrates is widely revered by contemporary societies for his highly regarded and selectively ignored Hippocratic oath. He is credited for shifting clinical thinking from mystical, ethereal, and magical ideas about what made people sick to more rational notions that disease could be explained by environmental and physical conditions. A singularly important Hippocratic observation of great relevance to Dr. Iatros' current condition is, "Our natures are the physicians of our diseases," referring to the fact that patients seemed to progress naturally with their illnesses, regardless of physician interventions (the modern-day observation of which seems to have precipitated the WADAO leading to Dr. Iatros' admission).

The Hippocratic tradition contains some key elements that have a significant role in Dr. Iatros' current illness:

- It closely tied physician diagnostic and therapeutic actions to the response of the patient (no more chanting, praying, and then embalming).

- It sanctified the relationship of patient and doctor, a responsibility that, in the estimation of medical historian Richard Gordon, "carried with it the core element that any nonphysician who attempted to direct the doctor's actions or practices, or interfered in any way with the doctor's singular devotion to patients, was not only inappropriate, but immoral."[18] This deeply ingrained professional dogma and attitude, combined with the fact that somehow physician actions should be directly responsible for how a patient fares, provides a strong foundation for resistance to suggestions about care from those outside the profession (such as case managers).

- It established the practice of collecting patient fees up front, with the amount being based on the patient's ability to pay and on sensitivity to the emotional effects a large fee might have on a tenuous patient. The patient's brother further relates that physicians in Hippocratic times were almost exclusively from aristocratic backgrounds and attended to upper-class patients, whereas physician assistants, apprentices, and slaves took care of the economically or politically disadvantaged and got to do the fancy diagnostic urine tasting.

- It generated the revered Hippocratic oath, which was not only dubiously adhered to in Hippocratic times but has been sketchily recalled by generations of family members up to present times. Select elements of the oath deserve emphasis because of their bearing on Dr. Iatros' current condition (and also because they point to Hippocracy):

  - The responsibility to keep patients from harm and injustice. (The origin of "above all else, do no harm.")

  - Application of measures for the sick, "to each by the best measures of my ability and judgment" (meaning, "I am at least in charge of you, if not the facts").

  - And the always remembered: "May it be granted to me to enjoy life and art, being honored with fame among all men for all time to come."

Medicine, Science, and Resistance

The patient's family history is rife with examples of difficulties with change, suggesting a heritable basis for inflexibility. Much of the resistance centered around difficulties in accepting science as a basis for medical practices. Even after the early application of science to medicine by the Greeks, the preferred approach of Byzantine and medieval doctors to illness remained based on the idea that disease was a punishment for a lapse from the purity of Christian life, and cure was solely the result of miraculous divine intervention.[19]

Decades after the discovery of bacteria by Louis Pasteur and the demonstration that diseases could be irrefutably tied to infectious micro-organisms by Robert Koch in the late 1800s, the physician family clung tenaciously to the concepts of mysterious "fomites," "miasmas" (arising in surgical wounds), and "particles of people" that modified themselves and spread to others as the causes of infection. Koch's famous postulates for demonstrating when organisms are the cause of a clinical illness represented early evidence-based medicine, a highlight in the family tree. These postulates and the concept of infectious disease later stimulated select members of the science family to discover and begin to prevent and treat many other illnesses caused by bacteria; protozoa; viruses; slow viruses; little bits of life called rickettsia; and, most recently, toxic infectious bits of protein called prions. But this lineage was very highly concentrated in the academic and scientific communities and was not very well accepted by traditional medical practitioners.

Physicians soundly rejected the concept of cleanliness as a factor in postoperative infections for many years, even though they were forced by science to grudgingly accept the idea there just might be infectious microorganisms.

Joseph Lister entertained the idea that something might be contaminating surgical sites (causing pus) some time before Pasteur and Koch proved the relationship between germs and disease, and he began swabbing and spraying operative sites with carbolic acid to cleanse them; his surgical colleagues thought he was being ridiculous. Physicians soundly rejected the concept of cleanliness as a factor in postoperative infections for many years, even though they were forced by science to grudgingly accept the idea there just might be infectious microorganisms. Mr. Gordon pithily notes that "sanitation in the operating theater was widely derided as finical and ladylike and affected, the equivalent of the block being scrubbed before use by a butcher or headsman."[20] Resistance to the notion of disinfection and antisepsis was accompanied by vociferous complaining by surgeons about the inconvenience of donning clean clothes or gowns rather than the pus and blood-stained jackets worn from procedure to procedure—the more disgusting the jacket, the more experienced the surgeon. (In 1890, rubber gloves debuted in the operating room, not to guard against infection, but to protect the hands of a surgeon's favorite scrub nurse from being stained by disinfectant.) It would be many years before gloving would be adopted, because the accessories were inconvenient and said to make it too hard to "feel" things in the operative bed. Later, in a fashion observable repeatedly in the Iatros family lineage, the practice of gowning and gloving would be carried to extreme, based on presumption rather than evidence. If a little is good and a lot is lucrative, a huge amount must be great.

While Lister was disinfecting, Ignaz Semmelweiss, an obstetrician in Vienna in the mid-1800s, was directing attention to hand washing. He observed that, in the two clinics delivering babies at the largest hospital in the world, three times as many patients died from child-bed fever (also called puerperal fever) on the ward where medical students attended the labor as did on the one where midwives delivered the children. He noticed how similar puerperal fever was to the disastrous disease medical students contracted when they cut themselves doing postmortem dissections in the anatomy lab, put that together with the fact that the medical students came to the labor decks directly from dissection (whereas the midwives never had such an honor), and deduced that child-bed fever must be due to something the doctors were transmitting to patients by sullied fingers.

Semmelweiss then did something unconscionable to prove his theory, something he had been influenced to do by a seedy character with whom he had studied in France—physician P.C.A. Louis. He gathered data, analyzed it, and thought about what was happening to the patients in light of it.

Based on his evidence, and over great hue and cry, he insisted on hand washing by students before attending deliveries, which reduced puerperal fever deaths on the students' ward from 18 percent to less than one percent. (This was 16 years before Pasteur and Koch demonstrated bacterial infectious disease and reveals the power of evidence, thought, and information in advancing human health, even when all the facts aren't yet known.)

In honor of his life-saving discovery and his well-intentioned mandate for hand washing, Semmelweiss was demoted by the chief of the hospital service, his practice privileges were limited, and his obsessive rules were condemned. Other surgical services, guarding their autonomy and confident of their practices, failed to institute cleanliness measures and completely rejected the idea of doing a clinical trial; his presentation to the Medical Society of Vienna was humiliatingly and viciously attacked. Semmelweiss went home to Hungary, where he again demonstrated the marked reduction in mortality associated with his simple hygienic procedures. After 10 years of making sure about all this, he published a book on prevention of child-bed fever, which was soundly rejected by physicians. Reduced to insanity and intermittently committed to lunatic asylums, Semmelweiss ultimately died from an infection, having cut himself during his final dissection.

Another striking example of resistance in the medicine family, which was joined by an anxious public, arose at the very start of the 19th Century in England. British doctor Edward Jenner, after 20 years of observing smallpox in his general practice, decided to use some pus from a cowpox sore on the hand of a milkmaid to vaccinate an eight-year-old boy, hoping to confer on him protection from contracting the full-fledged smallpox. (Several weeks after the cowpox inoculation, Jenner scratched live smallpox matter into the skin of the same James Phipps, finding happily that he subsequently developed no disease.)

Millions of humans had died of smallpox; it had decimated the Indian populations of the Americas, disfigured royalty in Europe, and led to a widespread practice of inoculation, consisting of taking pus from one individual with smallpox who looked as if they were going to survive and injecting or scratching it into the skin of a healthy individual. The usual result of inoculation was a mild case of smallpox from which the patient recovered, thereafter becoming immune to the more deadly form of the disease.

Jenner considered evidence that recovery from naturally acquired smallpox conferred immunity to both recurrent smallpox and to a more benign condition, cowpox. He observed that recovery from cowpox seemed to prevent contraction of smallpox, and asked himself: "Why not use less risky cowpox pus to confer protection from smallpox rather than the customary inoculation with smallpox pus?" A splendid example of an early risk/benefit analysis. The process of using a less toxic organism, such as the virus we now know causes cowpox, to confer cross-immunity to a more lethal but closely related organism, smallpox, is called vaccination. This was what Pasteur had been using on animals in France. The use of attenuated organisms, crippled or weak versions of the real infectious agent, is considered a type of vaccination as well. This was the process that inoculation really represented, because by the time the smallpox sufferer had turned the corner to survival and became a pus donor, the organism had been largely crippled by the survivor's natural immune defenses.

In honor of his life-saving discovery and his well-intentioned mandate for hand washing, Semmelweiss was demoted by the chief of the hospital service, his practice privileges were limited, and his obsessive rules were condemned.

The relevance of this discussion to Dr. Iatros' case, and the reason for the preceding detail is so one can appropriately ponder why Jenner's report on vaccination was soundly rejected by the Royal Medical Society, by physicians in practice, and by an inflamed public. As far as practitioners were concerned, anecdotal reports of vaccinated individuals metamorphosing into cows held as much sway as the scientific evidence in favor of vaccination.

Trench physicians fanned the fires of public disbelief, and the early rejection of Jenner's work by the "learned" medical establishment put quite the damper on the use of vaccination. An Anti-Vaccination League was founded that became influential in stopping free vaccination of English infants, eliminating vaccination of English children, and even halting vaccination of troops being sent into battle in France (so they could die by the capsids of a virus if not by the hands of the enemy). Napoleon, on the other hand, had his own son vaccinated for smallpox as an infant and encouraged a campaign for the vaccination of childen and army recruits. (This foresight left him with problems of typhus, hemorrhoids, and stomach cancer to deal with.[21])

In the end, however, after a miserable change process, mass vaccination spread, and, by 1977, smallpox was declared eradicated as a health threat from the globe. Happily, persistence and rectitude, and a late turnaround by the Iatros family, allowed a happy outcome in this specific area.

Science marched on and advances in pathology, physiology, anatomy, microbiology, and chemistry were forthcoming, but most members of the Iatros family evinced little interest in science-based innovations. Tools and practices of great value were slow to make their way into common clinical practice and generally met with knee-jerk resistance. Leopold Auenbruegger's method of percussion (the interesting thumping of the middle finger of one hand on the back of the middle finger of the other as it roams the back or chest, which emits different audible reverberations depending on whether fluid- or air-filled lung lies beneath the finger being tapped), which he had learned while checking out the fullness of wine casks at his father's pub, was one example. (This percussion technique was soundly rejected by Viennese doctors, who seemed to specialize in rejections. It was not until Napoleon's physician popularized the technique that it finally caught on in the year of the discoverer's death).

Trench physicians fanned the fires of public disbelief, and the early rejection of Jenner's work by the "learned" medical establishment put quite the damper on the use of vaccination.

René Laennec's stethoscope (a rolled up piece of paper in its inception) was another example. It was also René Laennec who solidified the ties of science to medicine in the form of some important principles. He insisted that physical changes in the organs of the cadavers he studied had characteristic relationships to pathophysiology; that signs of such changes in the organs could be observed and used to diagnose pathophysiology in the living, distinct from the more superficial disturbances or symptoms that accompanied an illness; and that conditions thus recognized should be treated uniformly in a way experience had shown was most effective.[22] He was, of course, largely ignored by family members for quite some time.

Anecdote and indoctrination were the basis of almost all medical rituals, and, with such "religious" teachings, it is understandable that resistance to adopting scientific methods was dwarfed in significance by failure to abandon ineffective remedies. Samuel Johnson astutely observed, "It is incident to physicians, I am afraid, beyond all other men, to mistake subsequence for consequence."[23] (I might add, "and then enshrine and teach the mistakes.")

> Samuel Johnson astutely observed, "It is incident to physicians, I am afraid, beyond all other men, to mistake subsequence for consequence."

One of the more remarkable examples of such a useless practice was "bleeding," which was adhered to with near religious fervor from Hippocratic times all the way to the early 1950s. Venisection (drawing blood by various methods of cutting veins) was modified and raised to an art form by French physician Victor Broussais, who found the idea of using symptoms to diagnose illness preposterous and treated just about everyone with heavy leeching and large doses of opium. He confabulated that draining off blood would selectively reduce the congestion observed in diseased intestines and elsewhere.[24,25] Benjamin Rush in America agreed with Broussais, insisting that letting blood and purging bowels was the universal cure for what he taught his students was "but one disease in the world."[26]

In the first quarter of the 19th Century, London imported on the order of seven million leeches annually for medicinal purposes from France, where three million per year were similarly used. To leech was to cure; it was the kinder, gentler way of bleeding patients, no more or less effective than cutting or suctioning, but somehow more chic. The efficacy of bleeding was a widely presumed medical fact. Any arguments about it had to do with how and whom to bleed, not whether to bleed. Broussais' techniques of applying blood-sucking leeches to patients; salting them to get them to perform better; and, in really tough cases, cutting off their behinds to get a steady exanguinating stream from the patient were widely accepted in France as opposed to the principles and diagnostic observations advanced by his contemporary, René Laennec, who was clearly on target but was getting no one to cotton to his findings.

Because diagnosing, recognizing, identifying, and naming diseases was not uniform, the rationale and the conditions mandating leeching were confused and predominantly a matter of opinion. In fact, the generally muddled way of observing illness, let alone recording symptoms and treatments for evaluation, detracted significantly from the ability to apply rational thinking to medical arts. Or so thought a spontaneous mutant in the Iatros family tree named Pierre-Charles-Alexandre Louis.

Louis, who studied medicine after first schooling in law, maintained the belief that detailed, precise clinical records on each of his patients (including their diseases, the effects of his treatments, and observations postmortem) should be collected and statistically analyzed, thereby contributing to a more solid understanding of diagnostic considerations and treatment efficacy. He persisted in tirelessly recording and accumulating, in a standardized way, detailed accounts on his patients, compiling enormous data files that he subsequently took a year off from practice to evaluate.

The results of his approach earned him the title "father of medical statistics" and allowed him to correctly describe the spread of tuberculosis, both within the tissues of individual patients and throughout populations. He applied his numerical approach to yellow fever and typhoid fever as well, with a precision that allowed typhus to later be distinguished from typhoid (caused by entirely different organisms), which in his time were seen clinically as a single disease. P.C.A. Louis is a less famous figure in the Iatros lineage, but his influence on others had enormous beneficial consequences for public health, which is really just the sum of individual health, when you think about it. It was he who put the first nail in the coffin of leeching, at least as far as its use in treating pneumonia, because the evidence he collected suggested its futility.

Because diagnosing, recognizing, identifying, and naming diseases was not uniform, the rationale and the conditions mandating leeching were confused and predominantly a matter of opinion. In fact, the generally muddled way of observing illness, let alone recording symptoms and treatments for evaluation, detracted significantly from the ability to apply rational thinking to medical arts.

This put a crimp in Broussais' style, but, because the medicine family was unable to incorporate change rapidly, the practice of bleeding waned only gradually over many years. Even as late as 1930, leeching was still recommended by some medical texts, but, by then, scientific understanding of microbiology and physiology had advanced to the point that alternatives were obvious. Of course, just because there was a better way didn't mean the old way was necessarily bad, or should be abandoned. One of the last and perhaps most satisfying application of leeches was in 1953 to a terminal Joseph Stalin, who had recently reminisced fondly about the four thousand officers he had "purged" from Soviet ranks and the torture and murder of his entire physician staff. In this case, the leeching (as a treatment for his cerebral hemorrhage) had its usual therapeutic effect.[27]

To summarize, the Iatros family tree reveals a marked tendency to ignore information, eschew change, decry the application of science to medical arts, defend anecdotally adopted methods, persist with ineffective practices long after they have been proved ineffective, and exaggerate and spread useful practices into areas where no proof of efficacy exists on scales for which there is no rationale. It also contains many shining examples of true thought-leaders who understood the importance of information, communication, rigorous proof of practice, and simple tenacity to scientific principles as weapons against disease.

Growth and Development

Much of Dr. Iatros' growth and development mirrors his lineage. Childhood reflected Hippocratic precepts in that more rational clinical thinking, observation, and reporting were learned and illnesses were recognized as having a natural rather than a mystical basis. This gave way in adolescence to a qualitative stage of medical practice, wherein structural changes in ill patients were tied directly to pathophysiology, with a shift from thinking about physiologic "humors" and diseases as entities emanating from the patient as a whole to an increasingly specific and localized understanding of illness. The new understanding fostered a growing expectation on the part of doctors and patients alike that, if enough investigation of enough "parts" was carried out with the new technology, a good doctor would be able to discover and fix just about anything. This comprehension gave rise to the principles of René Laennec mentioned in the family history section above. For purposes of illustration, recall that evaluating body substances as possible indicators of disease appeared early in Dr. Iatro's lineage. Tasting urine and noting its sweetness in diabetic patients was one example. Such inexpensive assessments gave way to measuring sugar levels in urine and later to detecting many substances in urine and other body fluids. This was a good practice when applied thoughtfully.

> Edward Tenner correctly surmised that, to better observe and evaluate focused "parts" of patients, technology was adopted that "revolutionized the way doctors saw, heard, and thought—and in turn changed the attitude of patients toward physicians and their own bodies."

In his insightful review of the effects of technology in a variety of areas of human endeavor, Edward Tenner correctly surmised that, to better observe and evaluate focused "parts" of patients, technology was adopted that "revolutionized the way doctors saw, heard, and thought—and in turn changed the attitude of patients toward physicians and their own bodies."[28] Some current medical ethicists see this development—the fragmentation of physician perceptions of the goals of medicine from success of the whole patient to outcomes for discrete parts—as the basis for present-day futile treatments.[29] Surgery, pharmacology, targeted therapy, and an improved understanding of pathophysiology emphasized evaluation of patients in pieces and parts.

Later in the 1800s, quantitative (measure something) methods were increasingly used to diagnose illness, further emphasizing disease explanations as malfunctions of subsystems within the complex human organism. The doctor-patient relationship shifted further from a fundamental nurturing one to one in which the physician was more of a technician, with modern tools and the ability to fix rather than support the patient.[30,31]

Measurements of physiologic function, such as temperature, blood pressure, and respiratory rate (the so-called vital signs) and other scientific discoveries allowed strides in the conquest of acute diseases (infection, local injury). It is arguable whether medical technologic advances in this developmental phase enhanced life-span or quality of existence, but what seems quite clear is that elimination of acute health problems made it more likely that patients would survive to become increasingly aware of chronic causes of suffering that were incurable by usual methods. (Doing for chronic illnesses what had worked for acute ones, but repeatedly and with greater intensity, seemed only natural, because there weren't any obvious alternatives.)

Substantial difficulties arose in the late quantitative stage of growth as new technology for detecting and measuring substances and for assessing parameters of health and illness exploded on the scene, starting Dr. Iatros down a disastrous road to excess. As the variety and the number of measurable parameters increased, microbiology and biochemical laboratories became indispensable accouterments of knowledgeable physicians, who used them as tools to gather data that then influenced their decisions. Frequently, however, there was little evidence of the utility of the new techniques and often no way to demonstrate in a scientific or systematic way either their superiority over clinical observation or their impact on the outcome of disease processes in the patient.

The range and volume of new tests quickly outstripped the ability of most practicing doctors to interpret them, let alone perform them personally; laboratory specialists evolved to conduct them and to determine what was normal or abnormal (absent most clinical facts altogether). At this point, Dr. Iatros entered a developmental stage in which decisions about patients relied on more than personal assessment and observation; he relied on data from others.[32] For a relatively brief time, science and technology appeared to be serving patients and doctors admirably, even though the doctors themselves were no longer in complete control of operations. In fact, even though the new tests seemed to distance doctors from patients, the collegial reliance of practitioners on each other around technology referrals was fundamental in creating the cohesive force that shaped the medical establishment in America.[33]

As Dr. Iatros matured, his dependence on the new technology grew, but his relative knowledge about its utility began to shrink. The technology fit well with the idea that disease was always due to a mechanical pathophysiologic problem, and it made sense that the more ways there were to test an ill patient, or screen a healthy one, the higher was the likelihood of finding a problem and providing relief.

In its early stages, simple direct testing generally led to a course of treatment based on results. Later on, however, testing became routine for confirming things, even when the diagnosis had been established by other means, and for excluding remote possibilities just to be safe. In America in the last half of the 20th Century, mortality rates did not change significantly, life expectancy did not elongate, new disease processes (with the exception of AIDS, which is still dwarfed in incidence by other causes of morbidity) were not discovered, and existing illnesses were not eradicated. The number of laboratory tests done per patient, however, more than doubled every five years from 1950 on. Worse yet was the practice of ordering things in a shotgun manner, searching for a clue rather than pursuing a logical course. As the number of tests on the menu increased rapidly, the probability of knowing what tests would be useful, and how, declined exponentially.

The doctor-patient relationship shifted further from a fundamental nurturing one to one in which the physician was more of a technician, with modern tools and the ability to fix rather than support the patient.

The range, complexity, and spectrum of these tests, not to mention early result inaccuracies and poor quality assurance, combined with the desire to avoid any doubt about a patient's disorder, pushed Dr. Iatros into the situation of reckless abandon. Exacerbating things were sloppiness and imprecision in recording the tests done, their results, the treatment choices made based on the results, and the ultimate effect of those treatments on the patient's condition.

Later on, however, testing became routine for confirming things, even when the diagnosis had been established by other means, and for excluding remote possibilities just to be safe.

Technology for imaging the human body was similarly abused, and because interpretation rather than measurement was part and parcel of most imaging studies, an additional human factor diminished accuracy. Multiple interpreters frequently disagreed on the meaning of the same image.[34] Determining the usefulness of an imaging procedure with respect to diagnosis, treatment, or long-term outcome was conveniently ignored for the same reasons that laboratory testing was exploited—lack of fiscal responsibility on the part of clinicians or patients, pressure to exclude all possibility of real or future illness, avoidance of lawsuits, ignorance, and profit.

Perverse incentives for testing were magnified when physicians were financial stakeholders in ancillary services. Doctors who owned laboratories ordered more than twice as many laboratory tests at a cost of $1 more per study on average than their same specialty colleagues without the conflict of interest.[35] The same phenomenon was demonstrated in medical imaging; physicians who referred to themselves for imaging on equipment they owned were four times as likely to obtain a study for a given symptom as were those who did not benefit financially from performing the procedure.[36] Physician groups that owned imaging equipment were almost twice as likely to use it to assess chest pain, four times as likely to use it to evaluate low back pain, and eight times as likely to use it to investigate knee complaints. When physicians owned an MRI unit, they used it 68 percent more frequently than nonowner colleagues to analyze low-back pain.[37,38]

Just as the cost impact of physicians' salaries was relatively insignificant compared to the explosion of expenses that was detonated by their decisions, so were the costs of malpractice premiums relatively small ($6 billion per year in 1988) in comparison to the expenditures that accrued to the practice of defensive medicine, wherein unnecessary tests or procedures were performed in an effort to avoid being sued (resulting in costs estimated to be between $12-15 billion per year).[39,40]

The barrage of tests and images meant that doctors knew more but comprehended less. (One insightful observer of society, Jeremy Rifkin, noted that high-technology culture in general seemed to divorce humankind from nature, giving us no real chance to become enlightened, as the word had been understood throughout history, and that our ancestors may have had less scientific understanding but perhaps a better intuitive grasp of what was really important in life.[41]) This technology run amok was a deadly development, particularly in combination with the lack of knowledge about the long-term value of a diagnostic test. Monetary incentives for technologists and providers of tests, added to the expectation that everything should be ordered and miraculously paid for whether crucial or not, lest one fall below the imagined ever-rising bar of standard practice, proved very problematic.

Monetary incentives for technologists and providers of tests, added to the expectation that everything should be ordered and miraculously paid for whether crucial or not, lest one fall below the imagined ever-rising bar of standard practice, proved very problematic.

As time went on, the lack of understanding about the impact of the testing on patient health (not to mention the harm that the tests could potentially cause), coupled with lack of consciousness about costs and resources, truly stunted Dr. Iatros' development. Compared to the enormous number of clinical decisions being made by every care provider on every patient, the amount of scientific evidence for the decisions was paltry; more testing was always better, and anything and everything that an individual or a group of doctors could think of to do for and to the patient, at any cost, was considered high quality and "consistent with the Hippocratic tradition." After five millennia of the individual physician as guardian of knowledge, the concept that there might be only one optimal valid way to diagnose or treat a disease was unfathomable.

Deeply troubling is the fact that, in this current phase of development, even when a wasteful process has been documented or pointed out to Dr. Iatros, he tends to react with the resistance that characterizes his ancestors. As a result, he has been hopelessly ineffective at trimming waste in many areas.

Sound evidence of many useless habitual practices and wasteful processes that have been pointed out to Dr. Iatros include routine neonatal umbilical cord Coombs and blood typing, prostate cancer PSA screening, routine preoperative laboratory tests, chest x-rays in general (but especially annual physical, screening, preoperative exams, and postvascular catheter placement or thoracentesis exams), upright abdominal films for abdominal pain, x-rays of the lumbar spine for low-back pain, ankle x-rays for sprains, bone radiographs for "healing" follow-up, pediatric abdominal x-rays for swallowed coins, skull x-rays for just about anything, x-rays of the tail bone or ribs for trauma, excretory urograms for hypertension, antibiotic prescriptions for nonbacterial illness, ritualized gowning in neonatal intensive care units, unnecessarily frequent changing of ventilator and respiratory tubing, needless and unrevealing sports physical examinations, tonsillectomy in children, and gastrointestinal surgery for peptic ulcer disease, to name but a few.[42-53] Taking action on the evidence, however, has been troubling, for reasons addressed below in the assessment portion of this consultation.

Education

It is important to review Dr. Iatros' education, because his current resistance to the application of scientific evidence in practice and to rigorous evaluation of his treatments seems to have some basis here as well as in his genes.

The roots of traditional medical schooling can be found in the same planter as those of formal clinical methods: the ever influential Hippocratic era. Although it is likely that passing folklore and magic from shaman to shaman was the general early rule (the Egyptian papyri notwithstanding), the nobility of empirical teaching was firmly established by the Greeks. The belief that the patient was affected by problems attributable to natural causes, rather than to anger of the Gods, gave rise to the thought that rational evaluation and reproducible therapeutic techniques should be applied. However, the incestuous teaching of family members—"here's my secret, pass it on"—free of charge, with admission by favoritism, may not have been so wise.

Hippocratic-age medical students learned by listening and watching more experienced physicians ply their trade in the field, helping with menial tasks and keeping equipment in top shape. Because there was no formal licensure, certification, or standardization and any male could elect to become a physician, finding a good physician in ancient times was likely a hit-or-miss proposition. The supreme value placed on "how to do this from my lofty and experienced viewpoint as the teacher, whom you will emulate, revere, and support, without disrespect or questioning until you call your own shots," however, seems to have been extremely resilient throughout the ages.

The years following Hippocrates are marked by enormous resistance to formal physician standards for learning, certification, and licensure. Debates raged over the propriety of mandatory education, the limitation of Hippocratic freedom to practice, and the appropriateness of nepotistic instruction. (One of the first attempts to formalize medical education was undertaken at a school operated in Edinburg as early as 1736. It subsequently took three successive separate Medical Councils, a General Council of Medical Education, and 160 years to finally set up orderly physician-certifying bodies in the British Isles.)

Dr. Iatros began his education in the United States in the late 1700s through apprenticeship and on-the-job training. As some "educated" doctors began to emulate their European colleagues by organizing medical schools and carving out specialties, hoping to elevate their status, they developed into a clique of sorts that came to be known as the "regulars" in distinction to lay practitioners using "folk remedies." The latter vastly outnumbered the regulars and claimed a right to practice medicine as an inalienable liberty comparable to religious freedom.[54]

By 1820, there were 12 or so private groups of doctors who had applied for state permission to teach and train physicians; in these early days of medical school, there was a nearly complete reversal of the Hippocratic methods—lectures were all there was for three to four months. Fees paid by students for this privilege were the sole source of sustenance for the schools, so it was pretty much a come all/graduate all enterprise. That was until the American Medical Association (formed in 1847) got involved, proposed lengthening the educational period to six

In 5,000 years of medical instruction and practice, standards of education have been enforced for only 0.18 percent of the total span.

months, and advocated more ethical rigor in student selection. Any schools that took these recommendations, increased entrance requirements, or increased workload during classes found themselves in deep financial trouble, because students would go to an easier or cheaper school or just set up practice without all the lecturing and learning.

As medicine began to organize and gather strength, the "regulars" enacted a code of ethics to furthur distinguish themselves from sectarian and untrained practitioners. As long as the "irregulars" were shunned by the regulars, they thrived. It was only after they were acknowledged by the medical establishment that they disintegrated, predominantly because regular medicine was producing demonstrable scientific results and advances, and alternative approaches were not.[55] By 1900, medical school education had advanced to the point that the president of Harvard University was moved to write: "The ignorance and general incompetenicies of the average graduate of American medical schools at the time where he receives the degree which turns him loose upon the community is something horrible to comtemplate."[56]

It wasn't until publication of the famous Flexner report on medical education of 1910, along with insistence by the AMA on quality classifications for teaching institutions, standardized testing, and certification that regulated medical education painfully arrived.[57] In 5,000 years of medical instruction and practice, standards of education have been enforced for only 0.18 percent of the total span. (As will be detailed in the assessment of this case, standards are not only relatively new to Dr. Iatros, but troublesome in many areas.)

By the mid-1800s, the explosion of knowledge in pathology, physiology, and pharmacology and the development of new technology (head mirrors, cystoscopes, x-rays, thermometers, sphygmomanometers, ophthalmoscopes, laryngoscopes, etc.) for doctors made it difficult for students of medicine to learn, let alone retain, new information. The new technology seemed to reduce dependence on patients' subjective accounts of their illnesses but increased dependence on equipment—and it definitely added "highly persuasive rhetoric to the authority of medicine."[58] When formal medical schools did arrive, some science, measurement, and statistical methods were taught, but the vast majority of clinical learning was still empirical; attending physicians and professors passed on experience, opinion, habits, and biases to fellows, residents, interns, and students.

Once in clinical practice, clinicians found themselves at a distance from new discoveries in medical science, and the insecurity associated with falling behind made them vulnerable to uncritical acceptance of nearly anything new that came along, particularly if it seemed to enhance or maximize care, provide new hope, or augment professional income.

Statistical evidence about the effectiveness of techniques or treatments was rarely sought and, if present but contrary to economic imperatives, was largely ignored.

The range and diversity of expert opinions, the absence of scientific foundation for intervention, and the imprecision of the language and methods taught in medical schools reinforced the notion that simply doing what one thought was best, based on whatever one had been taught, constituted high-quality care. Medical education still contains considerable folklore, and basic science that is taught is remarkably irrelevant in clinical practice.

Objective Findings

Vital signs —

- Blood pressure sitting and standing: 120/80; Temp. :98.6F
- Respiration: 12/minute; Pulse: 60/min., regular

Physical Examination —

- General: somber, asthenic but oriented, in no distress
- Head, eyes, ears, nose, and throat: normal
- Chest: unremarkable, no cardiac murmurs or signs of respiratory abnormality
- Abdomen: nontender, no masses
- Extremities: normal strength and motion
- Neurological: oriented to time, place, and position; memory normal; reflexes and strength symmetric and normal; gait normal
- Rectal: deferred
- (Complete physical examination to be performed on the ward by medical student)

Assessment

Dr. Iatros is suffering from a major depression, superimposed on narcissistic personality disorder, exacerbated by professional and financial psychosocial stressors. This primary diagnosis is complicated by severe informaciation with paradoxical data toxicity, infobia, and post-Hippocratic syndrome.

Major Depression and Narcissistic Personality Disorder

The somatic and behavioral elements of Dr. Iatros' illness, consisting of unhappiness, moodiness, insomnia, difficulty making decisions, fatigue, poor appetite and weight loss, and feelings of hopelessness, are all characteristic of depression. Most of the manifestations revolve around personal and professional disappointments, a sense of diminished stature, and frustration over loss of control over many elements of life.

Repeated damage to Dr. Iatros' self-esteem has occurred because of the unflattering revelations briefly mentioned in the history of the present illness. These problem areas bear elaboration, as they reveal that Dr. Iatros is not delusional or simply paranoid, but rather is aware of real difficulties, which is favorable for his prognosis.

Nearly two-thirds of controllable rising costs are due to increases in the volume and intensity of medical services (the content of care), which is determined by clinical decisions.

At the time of onset of symptoms (1975), Dr. Iatros' health care system was the third largest industry in the United States and was on its way to accounting for 11 percent of the country's gross national product. Insurance companies, government policies, and tradition had nurtured this growth, but things seemed to be getting a little out of hand as costs for care rose from $76 per capita in 1950 to $522 per capita by 1976.[59] (At this rate expenditures would exceed $1.5 trillion by the millennium.[60]) In 1991, when Dr. Iatros first presented in the emergency department, annual health care expenditures by payers exceeded $750 billion (a $76.8 billion jump from the preceding year.[61]) Health care remains the third largest U.S. industry, with half a million physicians, millions of nurses, and more than 5,500 acute care hospitals.[62] As of 1997, indications are that health care spending will continue to far outpace inflation, rising from $1 to $1.5 trillion per year.[63]

It seems the only parameter Dr. Iatros' family can agree upon, and routinely report in a standard way, is when a patient is dead.

At the time of this admission, the United States ranks first in the world in per capita expenditures on health care, nearly a trillion dollars per year. About 36 percent of the annual jump in spending is due to general economic inflation and another 9 percent to population growth. The other 54 percent of the rise is attributable to medical marketplace factors: 25 percent to rises in health care prices (wages, salaries, and overhead) and 29 percent to increased intensity of care (the number of tests, procedures, and treatments per patient visit.[61] Nearly two-thirds of controllable rising costs are due to increases in the volume and intensity of medical services (the content of care), which is determined by clinical decisions.[61,62]

The popular belief widely held by care providers and patients that these expenditures result in the best health care system in the world began to erode in the 1980s.[65,66] A 1984 Harris poll of satisfaction of Americans with provider interactions and hospital experiences suggested a changing attitude toward health care, indicating that fewer Americans were satisfied with their system than were the Canadians or the British with theirs.[67] Dr. Iatros was appropriately concerned that, despite the money being poured into the health care industry, the United States still ranked 25th among world nations with respect to infant mortality rates and failed to provide adequate health services to some 50 million people.[68] Despite what appear to be generally well-intentioned attempts at cost saving and quality improvement measures, and legislation intended to improve care coverage and services, the rate of nonelderly uninsured will be rising in 1997 from one in 6 to one in 5. Medicare fixes and equal care mandates such as the Kennedy-Kassebaum bill shift costs to private payers, resulting in large premium increases for everyone else.[69]

Infant death rates and population life expectancy are commonly used to compare national health programs, even though their lack of specificity and granularity make them quite subject to argument. Far more important than the comparisons themselves, and at the heart of the matter for Dr. Iatros, is the startling revelation that this is the extent of information available for assessing global health care practices. It seems the only parameter Dr. Iatros' family can agree upon, and routinely report in a standard way, is when a patient is dead. (Actually, there really isn't sound agreement even on this.[70])

Nonetheless, these gross indicators are somewhat illuminating. In 1990, the mortality rate in babies under one year of age was 9.1 per 1,000 in the United States, versus 4.6 per 1,000 in Japan, and life expectancy in America was 72 years for men and 78.8 years for women, versus 75.9 years for men and 81.9 years for women in Japan. In that same year, the United States spent 12.4 percent of its GNP ($675 billion) on health care, whereas the Japanese spent 6.5 percent of its GNP ($195.4 billion) for the same purpose.[71] While Japan was spending $1,113 per person to care for its entire population, the United States was spending $2,566 per person and failing to provide any services for some 30 million people, including 35 percent of the children who were not being immunized against childhood diseases.[71-73] Halvorson suggested that "we have the highest cost, lowest value health insurance system in the world, with the lowest percentage of people insured of any western country."[74]

Evaluators of the American system of health care pointed out that countries with better infant mortality rates than the United States were those that provided universal prenatal care for women, which was extremely influential in diminishing the rate of low-birthweight, high-risk babies. Instead of taking this preventive approach, at a cost of about $500 per patient, the United States focused on technologic "miracles" that were being achieved in newborn intensive care units, where very ill, drug-addicted, and premature babies were being saved at a cost of from $20,000 to $100,000 per child. It is painfully ironic that nearly half of all doctors practicing in neonatal ICUs are sued for malpractice, and nearly two-thirds of such practitioners have faced litigation if they have been in the specialty more than 15 years.[75] These same observers point out that a shift to optimum prenatal coverage could eliminate much of the need for neonatal intensive care, potentially saving $10 billion per year in the United States.[76-78]

Cardiopulmonary resuscitation (CPR), which was originally developed for patients with acute reversible or recover-able conditions, had become standard procedure for anyone who experienced cardiac arrest, regardless of disease or quality of life.

The beneficial effects of prenatal care on the outcomes of pregnancy were well established and accepted (even if not acted upon aggressively), but, in a fashion that typifies Dr. Iatros' style, there was no clear understanding of exactly how much prenatal care is needed to achieve good outcomes. If one could afford to see an obstetrician, 14 visits during gestation seemed like a fine round number. In low-risk pregnancies, world prenatal visit frequencies vary from a low of four (Switzerland) to a high of 14 (United States, Finland, and Sweden). Finally, a study has emerged suggesting that nine prenatal visits in uncomplicated pregnant patients, rather than 14, results in equally healthy deliveries and equally satisfied patients.[79] The next evaluation may indicate even fewer visits are necessary.

The same costly hypertechnical phenomenon is present at the other end of life's spectrum in America, with expenditures of billions of dollars to prolong unhealthy life in intensive care units rather than spending to promote healthy, safer life-styles.[80] There is no significant evidence that treatment in ICUs improves more lives than it harms; in one study of a surgical ICU, 54 percent of the patients died within a month of treatment and 75 percent died within a year, some from complications during treatment and others after needlessly prolonged, miserable, and undignified declines.[81,82] Cardiopulmonary resuscitation (CPR), which was originally developed for patients with acute reversible or recoverable conditions, had become standard procedure for anyone who experienced cardiac arrest, regardless of disease or quality of life.[83]

Between birth and death are some more granular statistics that have rightfully given Dr. Iatros pause to think. Nearly 80 percent of patients have ailments that will resolve on their own, without any tests, imaging, or treatment.[84] Thirty to 50 percent of expenditures in health care are for activities that produce little to no demonstrable benefit.[85] Only 10-20 percent of clinician actions are supported by scientific evidence of efficacy of action or treatment,[10] and, to a surprising degree, medical interventions are doing more harm than good.[86] To state it more gently, "physicians often do not quite understand how they arrived at the proper insight that put them on the right track to finding the correct diagnosis."[87]

Intrusions into Dr. Iatros' practice by outside forces to control costs were clearly warranted in the opinion of employers and other payers for care because of these revelations and because company health benefits expenditures had risen from 2.4 percent to 5.8 percent of compensation between 1970 and 1989, with a corresponding jump in health benefits from 23 to 36 percent of total benefits.[88]

Dr. Iatros' confidence and pride have been deeply shaken by these realizations; the ineffective and sometimes detrimental effects of the system in which he functions are exceedingly painful for him to acknowledge. He seems most bothered by inadequacy in the areas of medication, hospitalization, unintentional harmful results of care, and misuse of technology, which again points out that he is not delusional.

Medications ingested, inserted, or injected by some 80 percent of the American adult population everyday are of questionable effectiveness most of the time, and drug companies are spending as much on marketing products to overwhelmed doctors as they are on research (well over $6,000 per doctor per year); solid scientific proof of drug superiority and value are rarely part of the research and are never a reliable element of the "pitch."[86,89,90] Between 1981 and 1988, 84 percent of new drugs introduced were determined to work better than placebo (nothing) but not better than other drugs already on the market.[91] In one assessment of three anti-arrhythmic cardiac drugs, death rates were actually higher among patients randomly assigned to treatment with two of them compared to placebo, and effectiveness of the third drug was no better than placebo.[92]

To state it moderately, the cardinal element of the Hippocratic oath, to "do no harm," was being egregiously, if unintentionally, violated.

A recent study of antibiotic use in a pediatric Medicaid population for treatment of otitis media (where financial rewards for using more expensive preparations is not a factor) was very illuminating with respect to the costs of habits and misinformation. Where less expensive antibiotics were used as first-line treatment (amoxicillin, trimethoprim plus sulfamethoxazole or erythromycin plus sulfamethoxazole), fewer children required a second course of antibiotics as compared with those initially treated with more expensive drugs (ceflacor, amoxicillin plus clavulanate, or cefixine), and the adverse drug reaction rate was also lower with the less expensive drugs. The low-cost drugs, which were prescribed about two-thirds of the time, accounted for only 21 percent of total medication expenditures, whereas the more expensive drugs dispensed for the other one-third accounted for 77 percent of total expenditures. This means that if even half of the more expensive prescriptions could be replaced by the less expensive medicine in this population, effectiveness would rise, adverse reactions would drop, and a savings of nearly $400,000 would accrue to the system.[93]

Not counting unpredictable adverse effects, such as allergic reactions to drugs, it was estimated that one out of every 25 patients admitted to the hospital would suffer iatrogenic injury.

Further complicating the case of antibiotic drugs, which are clearly and demonstrably effective for specific infections, was the fact that indiscriminate use was resulting in resistant germs and complications (penicillin-resistant staphylococcus infections rose from 13 percent in 1960 to 91 percent in 1987).[94] U.S. hospitals were spending nearly nine billion dollars per year on antibiotics, and superinfection by microorganisms usually held in check by "good" bacteria that had been exterminated by the drugs was on the rise.[95] Patients were convinced by the medical establishment that antibiotics were wonder drugs, but they then assumed that, because antibiotics were so great for bacterial infection, they must be good for anything that felt like bacterial infection (colds, coughs, sinusitis).[96] Patients were receiving antibiotics for illnesses that were clearly viral or noninfectious in nature and on which the drugs had only a placebo effect.[97] Every year, some 10 million people visit clinicians for viral respiratory infections (colds), more than 90 percent of them leave with prescriptions, and more than half of the prescriptions are for ineffective antibiotics.[2]

The worry about antibiotic-resistant organisms and the future ineffectiveness of antibiotics against them seemed remote enough for Dr. Iatros to ignore, but adverse reactions to medicines of other kinds, and untoward interactions of drugs with each other, were more pressing. The trend of prescribing unproved medications and the results of their side-effects seemed to actually diminish the health of patients each year, and some researchers observed that secondary disorders caused by drugs ranked among the top 10 causes of hospitalization and killed more patients each year than cancer of the breast.[97,98] Fen-Phen is a recent notable blunder; thalidomide in the 1950s is perhaps the most notorious.[99,100]

Dr. Iatros was also aware that patients in hospitals weren't doing very well for their thousands of dollars per day. In fact, 20 percent of hospitalized patients wound up with doctor-induced illnesses as a result of their stay. Nearly 4 percent of admitted patients were actually being injured by hospital activities, half of which were due to physician error, and 14 percent of the injured actually died.[91,92] This was due, at least partly, to unnecessary operations, invasive tests, inappropriately pre-scribed medicines, and contagious illnesses contracted from other patients. Not counting unpredictable adverse effects, such as allergic reactions to drugs, it was estimated that one out of every 25 patients admitted to the hospital would suffer iatrogenic injury.[93] The black sheep of the family, Dr. Mendelsohn again rudely awakened care providers and patients to these problems by caustically contending that in hospitals, "if the drugs, the germs, the surgeons, the chemicals, or the accidents don't get you, you still stand a good chance of starving to death."[2] Also relat-ed to the adverse effects of hospitalization on health were humiliating reports that, when doctors went on strike for a variety of reasons in Israel in 1973, and in Bogota, Columbia, and Los Angeles in 1976, death rates in the effected communities went down anywhere from 18 to 50 percent. To state it moderately, the cardinal element of the Hippocratic oath, to "do no harm," was being egregiously, if unintentionally, violated.[2]

The use of technology in medical practice, which encompasses drugs, devices, medical procedures, surgical procedures, and supportive systems within which care is provided,[104] has been the quintessential element of Dr. Iatros' most recent developmental stage. There is little question that this technology, when appropriately applied, has improved the health and quality of life of many Americans. The problem, however, in times of diminishing resources, is that less technology use appears to have no deleterious effect on health status in countries such as England and Canada, where lower technology care is provided.[105] Even in hypertech-nical America, questions are arising about the efficacy of routine fetal monitoring in infant deliveries,[106] the appropriateness of routine obstet-ric ultrasound,[48] the utility of upper intestinal endoscopy,[97] the reasons for twice the number of CAT scanners in the United States than in other modern countries with similar health status,[108] and the wisdom of mass screening in a host of areas, just for starters.[109]

Although improved well-being, decreased mortality, and elongated life-span have been attributed to medical interventions, including treatment of infection, early cancer detection, and less complicated surgical tech-niques, greater life expectancy and diminishing mortality between 1900 and 1950 were largely due to improved nutrition and better sanitation, not to medical intervention. Sixty-eight percent of the reduction in bron-chitis, pneumonia, and influenza deaths; 90 percent of the decline in whooping cough; and 70 percent of the decline in diphtheria and scarlet fever occurred before the introduction of sulfa antibiotics in the 1930s.[110] After 1950, life expectancy leveled off and even began to drop, despite fab-ulous new medical technology.[111] When the proportion of the U.S. gross national product spent on health care began to skyrocket in the 1950s, nearly 92 percent of the decline in mortality for this century had already occurred.[108,112] A study conducted between 1960 and 1980 suggested that, even though sophisticated new diagnostic tools were becoming available, the rate of doctors' missing problems that, if detected, might have resulted in survival of patients actually rose from 8 to 10 percent.[113]

While medical costs were rising at twice the rate of inflation, diseases and illness due to societal and environmental factors (smoking, alcohol and drug abuse, violence, and accidental injury) were rising. Tenner, writing about the unanticipated revenge of technology in modern society, states the obvious in this regard when he notes that, in spite of all the medical technology, it was becoming clear that mechanisms of improved health were intimately connected to economic, environmental, and educational quality.[43,114]

"In 1986 we concluded that 'some 35 years of intense effort focused largely on improving treatment must be judged a qualified failure.' Now, with 12 more years of data and experience, we see little reason to change that conclusion....However one analyzes and interprets the data, the salient fact remains that age-adjusted rates of death due to cancer are now barely declining."

In 1900, the leading causes of death in the United States were influenza, pneumonia, tuberculosis, gastritis, heart disease, stroke, personal injury, chronic nephritis, cancer, diseases of early infancy, and diphtheria. In 1990, the rank order was heart disease, cancer, stroke, personal injury, chronic obstructive pulmonary disease, pneumonia, influenza, diabetes mellitus, suicide, chronic liver disease, and HIV. In 1900, the top five killers were *infectious* in origin; in 1990, the major causes of death were tobacco use, poor diet and activity patterns, and alcohol abuse.[115]

Anthony Kovner supports Tenner's remark, with the observation that Americans today, with 5 percent of the world's population, consume 50 percent of the world's cocaine, kill each other with firearms at a rate of around 19,000 per year, and include 25 million adults who cannot read well enough to understand a warning on a prescription bottle.[116]

At the time of Dr. Iatros' present admission, headlines have proclaimed a decline in death rates due to cancer for the first time since statistics started to be collected in the 1930s. The enormous amount of money accruing to diagnosis and treatment of cancer (nearly $100 billion/yr, according to the National Cancer Institute.[117]) has resulted in diminution of deaths from 135 per 100,000 in 1990 to 129.8 per 100,000 in 1995. A more critical look at the data, however, reveals that the age-adjusted mortality due to cancer in 1994 (200.9 per 100,000 population) was 6.0 percent higher than the rate in 1970 and that the effects of colossally expensive new treatments on cancer have been largely disappointing.[118] The lion's share of any changes, modest though they may be, is attributable to cessation of smoking and decreased human exposure to environmental carcinogens.[118] In fact, some researchers remark, "In 1986 we concluded that 'some 35 years of intense effort focused largely on improving treatment must be judged a qualified failure.' Now, with 12 more years of data and experience, we see little reason to change that conclusion....However one analyzes and interprets the data, the salient fact remains that age-adjusted rates of death due to cancer are now barely declining."[118] As emotional as death and dying are for human beings, the quality of life in "survivors" of cancer treatment is impossible to quantify.[119]

The individual needing attention is as accountable for decisions that influence his or her well-being as is the physician and is accountable for compliance with recommendations if they are soundly made.

Complicating Dr. Iatros' depression is the additional complexity of a mild form of psychological dysfunction called narcissistic personality disorder (NPD). NPD manifests itself in Dr. Iatros' confusion about real versus imagined power over disease. Its evidence has been repeatedly reflected in Dr. Iatros' heritage since antiquity and conspicuously fostered by societies that intermingled physicians with deities. Human beings have difficulty accepting their humanity, and physicians have difficulty accepting the limits of their power.[120]

It is worthy of note that the Hippocratic oath is sworn to Apollo physician and other gods, formalizing physicians as divine and elevating doctors to theological levels—confusion that seems to run as deep as spiritual thinking itself. In the minds and traditions of many practitioners, and in the expectations of their patients, is the belief that healers are somehow omnipotent and worthy of taking complete control of individual health decisions and processes. Most doctors are extraordinary people with compassionate intentions, but also with human failings; mistakes, while undesirable and of significant consequence, are inescapable.[121] Dr. Iatros and his patients have difficulty accepting the reality that clinicians, despite considerable learning, have limitations of cognitive recall, perceptual idiosyncrasies, biased thought processes, habitual tendencies, and reinforced resistance to change.

In the recent past, Dr. Iatros has been more comfortable addressing the personality problem as an ethical conflict. Whichever concept is accepted, the issue can be distilled to the tension between an individual patient's autonomy and responsibility for making decisions about his or her health and the deeply rooted medical tradition of the clinician as all-knowing caretaker. The Hippocratic positioning of the physician as chief or sole decision maker in affairs of health, and the accompanying shift of responsibility for health from the gods to doctors, leaves an important element of the works completely out of the picture. The individual needing attention is as accountable for decisions that influence his or her well-being as is the physician and is accountable for compliance with recommendations if they are soundly made. The lack of this sense of responsibility, as well as an attitude of entitlement to anything and everything medicine has to offer (in distinction to other forms of consumerism), is one major source of Dr. Iatros' problems.[43]

The more evidence that can be brought to discussions of diagnosis and treatment, the greater is the trust of patient in doctor (confidence) and of doctor in patient (compliance)

This tension is greatly aggravated by the fact that patients and doctors assume relatively little direct financial accountability for health decisions in the current health care system; patients feel entitled to medical services based on their popular or personal notion of what they need (demand for antibiotics for viral illness or x-rays for a host of reasons, for example) rather than on firm scientific evidence. From their perception, there is no cost, and they see no harm, and therefore withholding of unnecessary services by clinicians is perceived as cutting corners.

Dr. Iatros feels pressured to provide maximal, and sometimes even recreational, services (obstetric ultrasound to start the baby album) to keep his patients satisfied, and the assumption that the clinician is always in better command of the facts than the patient, and knows what is right, valuable, efficacious, or appropriate, is almost as dangerous as the assumption that the patient knows what he or she needs (see informaciation below).

The wisdom of engaging in shared decisions with patients, based on strong scientific evidence, does not mean that reliance on technology and preoccupation with business should be allowed to overshadow the less well-understood healing elements of compassion, trust, confidence, and caring in the doctor-patient relationship.

The ideal resolution to this conflict between patient autonomy and professional beneficence would be cooperative judgment, planning, and responsibility for health decisions between patient and doctor, based on clear understanding of the risks and benefits of interventions. It is imperative that Dr. Iatros encourage a shift from the style of professional beneficence (in which all care decisions are relegated to him) to one of greater patient autonomy (in which patients assume responsibility for their health and treatment choices).

Paul Starr explores the social and cultural elements of medical authority in his Pulitzer Prize winning look at the social transformation of American medicine. He cites the bonds between medicine and science, the priviliged status of scientific knowledge in the American belief hierarchy, and the natural vulnerability that accompanies sickness as the major factors in the ascendance and dominance of the medical establishment in our society.[122]

The wisdom of engaging in shared decisions with patients, based on strong scientific evidence, does not mean that reliance on technology and preoccupation with business should be allowed to overshadow the less well-understood healing elements of compassion, trust, confidence, and caring in the doctor-patient relationship. There is, in fact, evidence that psychosocial support and caring, in and of itself, may dramatically affect clinical outcomes.[123] The more evidence that can be brought to discussions of diagnosis and treatment, the greater is the trust of patient in doctor (confidence) and of doctor in patient (compliance) and the less need there is for cost control interdictions by third-party payers. Information and evidence can be gathered to support practices that are not high technology but are very effective. The quality of the interaction between the patient and the provider, the degree to which the patient feels the provider listened, understood, and provided adequate time for relating, is a contributor to compliance, treatment success, and satisfaction with care.[124] If Dr. Iatros could supplant the time and energy spent doing ineffective things with personal attention, kindness, and humane patient interactions, costs of care would decline, quality and health outcomes would improve, and customers would be much more satisfied.

The NPD also has a role in Dr. Iatros' feelings of rage, shame, and anger in response to criticisms of his practices. His expectation that his actions should always be worthy of praise, despite evidence to the contrary, causes him exaggerated discomfort. His sense of entitlement to reward and success and his desire for constant admiration have temporarily overwhelmed his ability to reason and grow in new directions. Dr. Iatros must realize that the position of honor and comfort he has enjoyed is a relatively recent phenomenon in America—doctors were not always the powerful authoritative professionals thay are today—and that the application of science and information to practice may be the only way to maintain this stature.

At the same time, however, there is much that Dr. Iatros feels bad about over which he has virtually no control and in light of which his anger is grandiose. He cannot control the attitudes of society or the ethical and philosophic constructs of the population he attends to. He cannot dictate whether maximal care for the individual should supersede optimal health for the community, or magically solve environmental or social causes of morbidity. He cannot eliminate the picketing extremists who publicize or politicize what should be deeply personal medical decisions, regardless of their nature.

Depression, narcissistic personality disorder, and stresses that have been reviewed up to this point appear to have a unifying root cause: *inadequate information upon which to base clinical decisions and to conduct activities.* This information paucity can be considered in three categories for clarity, although they are virtually inseparable: severe informaciation (with paradoxical data toxicity), infobia, and post-Hippocratic syndrome.

Severe Informaciation

Dr. Iatros suffers from problems in communicating, collecting, and analyzing clinical information. Methods of documenting care are poorly organized and records are often inaccessible at the time of care delivery.

Because paper-based documentation has stagnated for in 5,000 years, critical facts are unavailable to the physician at least a third of the time when decisions must be made.

The emphasis on empirical methods, culturally and educationally, over many generations has fostered divergent practices based on emotional experiences "in the trenches" (see post-Hippocratic syndrome below), and this same diversity exists in the words and concepts Dr. Iatros uses to record care. The lack of standard descriptions has made the application of scientific rigor to the art of medical practice and to review of outcomes of medical interventions extremely difficult. Finally, data collected on the basis of billing codes are inherently biased and suspect because of subjectivity and manipulation for purposes of maximizing remuneration; therefore using them to determine quality of care is dangerous.

Present problems in the diagnostic category of informaciation therefore fall into three areas:

- Inadequate patient information when clinical decisions are made.

- Inadequate evidence to guide diagnostic and treatment choices and to maximize effectiveness and value.

- Data toxicity: an overload of redundant, inaccurate, uninfomative, or confusing facts, leading to incorrect conclusions.

Inadequate patient information at the time of decision making

Dr. Iatros' patients often require services at multiple physical sites and in various settings. Because paper-based documentation has stagnated for 5,000 years, critical facts are unavailable to the physician at least a third of the time when decisions must be made.[125] This is true in emergency department nearly 100 percent of the time, when prior health information is most important. In small private office practices, the paper medical record may be complete as far as the individual provider is concerned, but little or no information about the state of the patient's health or disease episodes outside of that specific office is reliably available, particularly when such care was delivered at a hospital. Hospital records, which began as sketchy entries in institution logs, gradually evolved into journals of mixed, unrelated events with minimal utility beyond day-to-day review of findings, comments, administrative detail, and staff communication.[126] They are rarely if ever meaningfully connected with the "longitudinal" health history, because individuals are not identified by a national unique health record number that would allow coalescence of their care records.

Outpatient paper records were and still are disorganized, illegible collections of personal notes variably recorded data and sundry test results.[115] Information is often missing or inaccurate, and the loose format and fragmentation of information impedes searchability and defies logical grouping of problems.[126] The lack of standard format, content, language, and completeness makes retrieving information from such records difficult, and what can be harvested is often of dubious value.

The problem-based progress note, introduced in 1970 by Dr. Larry Weed (and variably exercised), encourages more organized charting.[128] The SOAP (subjective, objective, assessment, plan) format followed in this case documentation logically segments information, at least placing things in standard groupings, but it has done little to improve the medical chart as a whole.

Even if medical records could suddenly become complete, legible, and uniformly available, Dr. Iatros faces a very serious problem that stems from a lack of standards for using clinical terms and concepts.

In larger integrated care programs, where inpatient, outpatient, primary care, and specialty care are provided in a coordinated single system, a more complete health record may exist for member patients, provided they have received their treatment within the "system," but getting the paper record to providers at the moment of care is inhibited by the need for physical transport. This limitation of access nullifies many of the benefits that should accrue to integrated delivery systems, fosters duplicative testing, and necessitates work-ups and hospitalizations that might have been avoided if the records were present.

Because uniform relevant structure is often lacking in the paper records, finding, reading, and interpreting the scribbling lowers confidence in completeness and accuracy. Diagnostic, therapeutic, medicinal, historical, examination, health risk, and prevention-related information is disbursed randomly through the medical record, at the whim of the documentor or of the medical records clerk. Illegible writing, arcane acronyms, personal cryptic abbreviations, and misfiled information are the rule.[125] The time needed to retrieve and decipher the information, when it's there to be found, is enormous, consuming the physician's most valuable resources, time and thought.

The ability to access vital information has fallen farther behind as fragmentation in continuity of care has progressed. Increased ambulatory services, a more peripatetic population, and fluctuation in doctor-patient relationships when alternate health plans are selected by employers all contribute to dispersal of individual records. The waste inherent in the antiquated system of recording and communicating clinical information contributes largely to Dr. Iatros' inefficiency and flawed judgment. The costs of requesting needless tests or of making poor clinical decisions because patient data are unavailable are enormous, not to mention the secondary ramifications of repeating potentially harmful activities. Because these unacceptable records are also used by members of the legal profession as official evidentiary documents of care, it is little wonder that Dr. Iatros feels helpless and victimized and that he fears litigation for incorrect decisions.

The unstructured, chaotic terminology used to document patient care in medical charts makes evaluation of aggregated data across a health care system or a panel of patients nearly impossible.

Even if medical records could suddenly become complete, legible, and uniformly available, Dr. Iatros faces a very serious problem that stems from a lack of standards for using clinical terms and concepts. Failure to agree upon uniform language and descriptions (in the useful fashion of Linnaeus' classification of life forms, for example) has severely hampered Dr. Iatros' ability to apply science to treatment. Whereas scientists start with well-thought-out conventions, for the most part, and adhere to them in the interest of advancing knowledge, medicine developed few such conventions as it dragged itself from the mire of mysticism. Even reliably reproducible anatomic structures have borne multiple diverse and aggrandizing eponyms; terms for diseases, tests, and findings are as variable as the multitude of physicians who report them. Geographical vernacular, idiosyncratic jargon, synonymy, abbreviation, and personal patterns of expression are the norm. The immediate consequence of this "free expression" is diminished quality of clinical communication, but the more damaging effect is examined next.

Inadequate information for establishment of evidence-based practice

The unstructured, chaotic terminology used to document patient care in medical charts makes evaluation of aggregated data across a health care system or a panel of patients nearly impossible. The lack of uniformity, recoverability, and comparability of information from chart to chart and from provider to provider, and the time and effort required to recover analyzable data, have been potent inhibitors to performing appropriate investigations of costs, benefits, and outcomes of treatment.

The advent of computing and information systems has magnified the deleterious nature of Dr. Iatros' lack of lexical standards. Now that new technology that can allow him to discover and prove his effectiveness and to demonstrate value is available, he is rendered impotent by the paucity of meaningful, comparable grist for the high-tech mill. Much of the ambiguity, redundancy, and confusion (over a hundred terms for hypertension, for example) exist because experts prefer to bicker rather than agree and because idiosyncratic medical culture has reinforced diversity (and the challenge of a good fight) rather than agreement or methodological evaluation. Imagine the confusion that would result if a relatively large and diverse group of geographers was allowed to name cities any way it preferred, without a mandate for agreement on the name within the group and with no prohibition against using the same name for multiple cities or different names for the same city. Medical terminology often functions as an elitist jargon that elevates the clinician's image of erudition in the eyes of the masses, who assume, incorrectly, that doctors actually understand one another.[2]

Unfortunately, this pool is now being exploited by businessmen, entrepreneurs, and health care bounty hunters to strip costs from a fat system, with little attention to the effects of such methods on patients (and little return of profits from the activities to the patients).

Laudable attempts to cross map, catalogue, and unify medical terminology have been made, and multiple "right" clinical vocabularies have been introduced.[129] They have resulted in proprietary and diverging sets of standard terms.[130] To use a relevant historical analogy, practitioners are leeching while arguments rage about whether it's "leeching," "bleeding," "cupping," "venisecting," or "phlebotomizing"—as if terminology made any difference in the effectiveness of the technique.

Dr. Christopher Chute of the Mayo Clinic suggests that "improvement of medical knowledge about best practice depends upon the ability to study practice outcomes and apply them to the patients we see. This implies that we can generate data about our patients that is comparable, so that it can be used in aggregate analysis, and so clinical decision support resources can be linked to patient data in real time. The single greatest obstacle to comparable data remains medical terminology. Failure to adopt and embrace a common terminology will doom outcomes research and data-driven clinical guideline development."[131]

Dr. Iatros' failure to develop and use clinical information systems designed by clinicians for patients has made him vulnerable to those with less knowledge but more data.

The medical education tradition has only made the terminology issue worse, because it promotes verbiage based on personal experience without standard agreements. Terminology finds its way into well-accepted medical textbooks, just as do opinions and anecdotes, despite the fact that they are unsubstantiated by scientific or epidemiological studies. Once in such tomes, these words, anecdotes, and observations are often referenced by the legal system to establish a standard of care, adding insult to injury.

Dr. Iatros is likely to fall further and further behind unless he adopts technology that provides complete information on his patients, along with factual evidence to support his judgments whenever possible. This means that results of outcome studies, risks and benefits of innovations, costs of tests or treatments, protocols for work-up and timely, and updated evidence-based practice guidelines must be made available to caregivers via the same instruments they use on an ongoing basis to record their clinical activities. (These "just in time," succinct information flashes have already been shown to be useful in eliminating wasteful activity and in modifying behavior.[132-136]) All of these capabilities depend on standards in terminology and on equivalency and comparability of terms.

Paradoxical data toxicity exists in at least two forms for Dr. Iatros. The first is the ambiguous, biased, or incorrect information that has been based on billing codes. These codes, leveraged for unintended purposes, have been accepted uncritically because they are intended for financial purposes, not clinical wisdom or truth. They fall far short of clinical accuracy; are often contaminated by code creep, unbundling, ambiguity, imprecision, and sloppiness; and have resulted in a virtual swamp of polluted data.[125,126] Unfortunately, this pool is now being exploited by businessmen, entrepreneurs, and health care bounty hunters to strip costs from a fat system, with little attention to the effects of such methods on patients (and little return of profits from the activities to the patients). Dr. Iatros' failure to develop and use clinical information systems designed by clinicians for patients has made him vulnerable to those with less knowledge but more data.

The second form of paradoxical data pollution results when facts associated with a patient or a condition fail to meet the criteria of information and become red herrings, noise, or diversions from more relevant issues. Often referred to as false positive or false negative results, they essentially amount to obfuscating garbage, which generally encourages further expensive test ordering to sort them out, resulting in a quagmire of burdensome data. Information is distinguished from data in that it must be comprehensible and useful to the person who needs it, available when it is needed, and accurate in the sense that the same data aggregate always equals the same information (some call this validity). It must contain all of the data necessary to make the user confident that it is complete. It must be concise and clear, and it must be comparable to other instances of the same information, with the same precise meaning.

The informaciation is a very serious condition for Dr. Iatros, because it prevents him from discovering what is right in treating his patients. In the present resource-constrained environment, clinical information systems represent the only realistic method Dr. Iatros has to mitigate misuse of tests, balance biases inflicted during training, validate or disprove community standards, and avoid the natural human tendency to make damaging emotional judgments about care.[139] In order for Dr. Iatros to make proper decisions and take more effective actions to benefit his patients and the health of his community, he will clearly need to know more about information systems and feel comfortable and competent using them. This need brings to light the next diagnostic consideration.

Infobia

Infobia refers to the combination of two powerful fears: fear of appearing incompetent using information system technology, and fear of the potential harmful effects information might have on position, prestige, or job security. Infobia is observed in Dr. Iatros' responses to my question about information system use in the History of the Present Illness. (Anyone who has worked to gain widespread physician acceptance of computer systems for use in patient care can attest to this issue.) Infobia exists in other types of care providers, and in workers in nonmedical fields to varying degrees, but it seems particularly rampant and severe among the Iatros family.

Physicians are held in high esteem, and the criticisms and foibles pointed out so far do not diminish the critical role they have in society. They can cure disease, maintain health, relieve pain, intervene in

Medical professionals may dispute some of the contentions of this case presentation, but few would deny that clinical practice is an enormously information-intensive process and that having information is critical to appropriate diagnosis and treatment.

suffering, and contribute to community on a deeply human level in ways that have no equal in other professional practices. To attain this stature, doctors undergo some of the most brutal training that can be dispensed: sleep deprivation, humiliation by superiors and uncontrollable emergency situations, guilt because of inadvertent or unavoidable errors, inordinate pressure to recall facts and react quickly to sudden dire situations, and stress from having to make critical decisions without complete information.

Medical students are as adequate as they can be, but they are still relatively incompetent. Interns are less than competent too, as are residents and fellows. Inexperience is a natural component of education, but, in medicine, the consequences and fears and stress around this process are very intense. Some people deal with this stress better than others, but none escape it.

Physicians are held in high esteem by society, and the criticisms and foibles pointed out so far do not diminish the critical role they have in society. They can cure disease, maintain health, relieve pain, intervene in suffering, and contribute to community on a deeply human level in ways that have no equal in other professional practices.

There may not be a worse experience than medical training, short of combat, for which one can volunteer. It is little wonder that, by the time they have endured medical school and residency, physicians have a very visceral reaction to the concept of being or seeming to be incompetent ever again. In fact, fear is probably the major lasting component of medical education; doctors are terrified of making a mistake or missing a diagnosis, worried about potential negative or unflattering comments about their ability by other practitioners, frightened of being sued, and extremely anxious about being afraid. Dr. Mendelsohn points out that "to hide their fear, they're taught to adopt the authoritarian attitude and demeanor of their professors."[2] The more terrorizing and fatiguing the training, and the greater the possibility of catastrophic error on a moment-to-moment basis, the more likely it is that the effected individual will later find change intolerable and more vigorously cloak him-or herself in the arrogance that confers a sense of safety.

There is a deeply rooted, painfully incorporated desire not to appear incompetent in front of patients or colleagues, no matter what benefits may ultimately accrue. Medical professionals may dispute some of the contentions of this case presentation, but few would deny that clinical practice is an enormously information-intensive process and that having information is critical to appropriate diagnosis and treatment. Placing a computer containing a patient medical record in front of a physician in the examination room, however, is likely to engender a kind of terror and rage reserved only for the most egregious of atrocities. (This reaction has mollified in recent years as the technology has become more user-friendly and common and there are some medical professionals who rely on some information systems frequently, but the reluctance serves to illustrate the key point.)

Within medical specialties, procedural technologic advances, such as laparoscopic surgery and stone lithotripsy, are generally well received (and then overused). There is usually a mild initial fear of change and of temporary incompetence. This is overcome rather quickly, because the technology in question contributes to the esteem of the medical professional; not many patients can criticize a physician's clumsiness in passing the scope, because patients don't know how to pass a scope, but the average grade school child today may have greater computer savvy than the average doctor. The triumph of "Big Blue" at the chess table in 1997 makes professionals in medicine understandably nervous when they read that a computer program applied to chest pain patients in emergency departments was slightly better at accurately excluding heart attacks than physicians and equally as good at diagnosing them; if the computer replaced the doctor, ICU admissions would have dropped 11.5 percent, resulting in significant savings.[140]

In considering and managing Dr. Iatros' infobia, it is important to interpret the reasons that computers in the examination room, no matter what important information they provide, have been so resolutely rejected by him:

- "I can't type." (Infobia translation: "I will appear incompetent as a typist, even though I typed 245 term papers as a student.")

- "Typing is for clerks." (Infobia translation: "I couldn't possibly be less competent than a lowly clerk.")

- "I need to be warm to my patients in order to heal, and technology interferes with my human touch" ("Except when this scope is half way up the descending colon.")

- "I can't see patients as quickly if I have to use this computer" ("I'd prefer someone else to spend half their time searching for information.")

- "If you give me all that information every time on every patient, there is no way I will be able to read it anyway" ("I only want what I want, and only I know what that is.")

The arguments point to the fact that Dr. Iatros has an intense desire never to return to the psychologically painful time and state when temporary incompetence was so agonizing. This phenomenon, in varying degrees, is common to all humans, who, when asked to change or adopt something new or let go of something old, automatically experience the "I'm going to feel bad again" recollections of the past. Those particularly effected by extreme hatred of change or of anything new are exhibiting an entity called "mosoneism,[141] which is mentioned only to provide you with a new and very applicable term with respect to change in medicine.

The other face of infobia in medical culture is also a byproduct of the medical education process, because the painful training installs belief in professional autonomy and empirical methods rather than in agreement and statistically valid evidence. Guidelines and protocols, therefore, may be viewed as anti-Hippocratic constraints, implying restriction of independent judgment. Just as, in business management circles, judgment and wisdom and sometimes intuition are extremely highly valued, definition, measurement, and exposure of the actual effects of medical interventions, while clearly the right thing to do, can be enormously troublesome for practitioners who hold this value sacred. Tenner suggests: "They fear, probably rightly, that computerized norms will rob them of professional discretion and initiative."[142]

Caregivers have a very understandable reason to be wary of the validity and vagaries of data collected with respect to practices so far, but it is interesting that absent data are more acceptable than some data. This fascinating rationale seems to suggest that ignorance is a valid reason to continue comfortably doing what has always been done, rather than risk illumination that mandates change.

Like professionals and workers in nonmedical fields, clinicians are concerned that bad or incomplete information will be used against them. In fact, the most troublesome issue is that new information will almost certainly dictate elimination of many customary practices; both patients and providers may view such changes as a loss (in attentiveness for patients and in income for clinicians) no matter how important it may be to do the right thing.

If good information is not gathered and evaluated within the health industry and presented to clinicians in the form of helpful guidelines, and if caregivers cannot convince themselves and their patients that the changes are not losses but gains in quality, legislators, employers, and other outsiders will make bad and arbitrary decisions for economic reasons to the detriment of all. Even so, analyses of which medicines are effective in light of their cost, which diagnostic tests have value to the patient's health, and which clinical interventions scientifically effect outcomes place a rather hard, cold vise on traditional medical methods.

Culture, values, beliefs, reward systems, and habit determine the ability of professionals to change, which brings me to the last important diagnostic consideration in this case.

Post-Hippocratic Syndrome (PHS)

PHS refers to the peculiar adherence to select teachings, precepts, social entitlements, and educational methods inherited from ancient Greek ancestors, while at the same time selectively "forgetting" others in a fashion that is significantly maladaptive and unbalanced in the modern world. The syndrome is very difficult to distinguish from informaciation. (PHS is misleadingly named, because many of its elements antedate Hippocratic methods and writings.) A complete review of PHS and its many manifestations might be counterproductive, in that it would stir up social, political, and pseudo-philosophical issues that could digress from the case at hand. The discussion therefore will remain focused on only the essential damaging elements:

- Adherence to the doctrine of professional beneficence and the treatment of each patient based on individual physician ability and judgment (the Hippocratic oath swears to "my" judgment, and makes no mention of the patient's role in a medical decision) as an excuse for failing to seek out or heed scientific evidence (of which there was precious little in 400 BC).

- Adherence to sanctification of the relationship of patient and doctor, implying prohibition of outside scrutiny of practice.

- Adherence to anecdote, empirical, and folkloric methods of medical knowledge transfer, with reverence for provincial teaching.

- Adherence to entitlement of honor and fame as a given, by virtue of membership in the profession (which in the oath is predicated on compliance with all of its proscriptions).

- Selective amnesia for suggestions about preventive medicine, societal ethics, diet, hygiene, and health maintenance as physician duties.

- Selective amnesia to a familiar laudable lament of the Hippocratic oath, to do no harm, which is manifest in unintentional but omnipresent iatrogenic illness or injury.

- Selective amnesia for Hippocratic dictums to base fee collections on patient financial status, with sensitivity to the potential adverse effects of such fee collection on the patient's health (perversely encouraged by the concept of "insurance").

The "Hippocratic tradition," reinforced by educational practices that have long elevated judgment, ability, and opinion above constructs of scientific proof is the most significant aspect of Dr. Iatros' current problems.

End-to-end evaluation of the chain of events from diagnosis to outcome and of costs and benefits at each step of testing and treatment along the pathway is very important yet virtually nonexistent in current practice.

End-to-end evaluation of the chain of events from diagnosis to outcome and of costs and benefits at each step of testing and treatment along the pathway is very important yet virtually nonexistent in current practice.[10] The absence of information and evidence of efficacy, combined with relative blindness to risks that attend virtually any medical intervention, has convinced Dr. Iatros and his patients that any action of possible benefit should be done. The following important pathway examples are presented to demonstrate the breadth and depth of this problem for Dr. Iatros and to emphasize the importance of information and information systems in his treatment.

Laparoscopic cholecystectomy nicely demonstrates an improvement in a step in a pathway, in that new technology allows removal of the gall bladder with less cost and morbidity. Patients needing cholecystectomy are fortunate indeed for the innovation. The problem with the pathway as a whole, however, is that the less invasive procedure is used more extensively than necessary (by as much as 50 percent in one study), actually raising the overall costs of gall bladder disease management by as much as 11 percent, not to mention the risks and pain of applying the procedure to patients who would not have been candidates for cholecystectomy based on signs and symptoms before the advent of laparoscopic surgery.[143] Evaluation of the entire gall bladder disease pathway, with assessment of costs, complications, and outcomes, and comparisons of laparoscopic surgery to traditional surgical cholecystectomy, nonsurgical treatment, and no treatment is difficult because of inconsistencies of data, sloppiness of language, and other manifestations of informaciation. The same phenomenon is seen with many other new less invasive techniques (catheterizations, arthroscopy, and gastrointestinal endoscopy are examples) that have been rapidly diffused into practice in the United States without careful consideration of their superiority to existing measures or of their cost efficacy.[144]

Despite these three factors that suggest limited, directed use of chest radiography, it became an accepted, expected, and in many instances standard of care examination, even when patients had no complaints referable to the chest.

A striking example of how this phenomenon can be expanded to epic proportions by legislators is seen in the results of the Medicare End-Stage Renal Disease (ESRD) Program enacted in 1972. The congressional act provided universal access to dialysis or transplantation at no cost and with no limitations to individuals with end-stage renal disease. This seemed reasonable and well-intentioned for patients in whom ESRD was the only or the overriding health issue. The problem was that, with financial barriers removed, patients who were never envisioned to be dialysized or transplanted (including those with multiorgan failure and severe systemic disease) started receiving frequent regular dialysis, resulting in a mere $6 billion per year cost overrun.[145]

This kind of confusion is a sure sign that something is awry.

PHS entitlements and precepts protect the right to deliver and charge for steps in the pathway as long as the doctor recommends them and the patient desires them (provided the cost diffuses unnoticed into the economic atmosphere). Because monetary rewards for the clinician and the perception of more as high quality by the patient are the norm, interesting routine and screening procedures have been propagated throughout the land. As a general rule, any activities preceded by the word "routine" or "screening" require immediate end-to-end analysis.

Although there is some evidence that screening identified segments of the population for disease to which they are at high risk improves quality of care and yields financial benefits of early disease intervention, indiscriminate preventive mass screening in the general population does not appear to lower cost or provide improved quality.[109]

Chest x-ray administration (also called chest radiography or chest roentgenography) and mammography illustrate some of the problems associated with injudicious disease detection schemes. Chest x-rays, which are the most common radiographic study performed (at a cost of some $11 billion per year presently), were accepted and promulgated largely on the basis of faith, anecdote, and expectation.[146] It was extremely interesting to be able to peer inside the human body with magic rays in the early 1900s; there was a sense of wonder and power as images confirmed diagnoses and made new significant and incidental findings.

The adverse physical and psychological effects that accompany false positives are generally underestimated; worry, fearfulness, psychological barriers to appropriate care, stress, pain, and complications from attempts to prove a finding inconsequential are, well, consequential.

As time went on, however, three things became apparent. First, as Sir William Osler observed, "in the majority of cases the x-ray tells us no more than a careful clinical examination."[147] Second, there is a very high rate of interobserver disagreement over radiologist findings and of errors (20-50 percent) in interpretation (over 50 million errors per year today).[34,148,149] Third, there is a small but definite risk of harming health associated with exposing patients, and in particular their reproductive (gonads) or rapidly dividing (thyroid, bone marrow) tissues to low doses of ionizing radiation, of which x-rays are one type.[150]

Despite these three factors that suggest limited, directed use of chest radiography, it became an accepted, expected, and in many instances standard of care examination, even when patients had no complaints referable to the chest. The more available radiographic equipment became, the less apparent the cost of a chest x-ray to the patient (thanks to insurance), and the more lucrative the unnecessary procedure for the provider, the more entrenched the procedure became in health assessment.[146]

Many of the more routine uses of chest radiography have recently been debunked (preoperative chest x-rays, cancer screening chest x-rays, and smoker chest x-rays, for example), although they continue to be done by many unenlightened providers.[151-153] The impact of chest radiography on the outcomes of disease and treatment has never been studied.[154] (This is not to suggest that chest radiography is not valuable and useful in specific cases; Dr. Iatros just doesn't know exactly what they are.)

Of the long line of dubious screening techniques for early detection of cancer that have been promoted, mammography may be one of the most troublesome examples, because breast cancer has such emotional significance and because the procedure itself has been heavily sold to and accepted by nearly every practitioner and woman in America. Several organizations (American College of Radiology, American Cancer Society, National Institutes of Health, American College of Obstetrics and Gynecology, and United States Preventive Services Task Force) have had frequently revised and differing recommendations, ranging from mammograms in all women with breasts (and some without) to women only in certain age groups, to women in certain age groups with specific risk factors, to all women with breast abnormalities on physical examination, to select women without physical examination findings, each recommendation with different intervals and frequencies. This kind of confusion is a sure sign that something is awry.

While very confused mammography factions fight out the age at which screening should begin for women (the debate rages publicly in popular periodicals), one courageous evaluator in this area, Dr. David Plotkin, has made a number of very interesting observations and eloquently joined the ranks of those who have quietly suspected his ideas are right for some time. After careful consideration of the studies that have been done and of their inherent limitations and biases, he points out that the death rate from breast cancer in 1992, despite expensive improvements in anesthesia, surgical technique, mammography, radiation and chemotherapy, bone marrow transplantation laboratory testing, and medical imaging, was 26.2 per 100,000 women; in 1935, before all this, the rate was also 26.2 per 100,000 women.[155,156] (The age-adjusted death rate due to breast cancer in American women for 1993 was determined to be 25.9 per 100,000 by the NCI, but drops in deaths here and in Great Britain are more likely the result of widespread, more effective tamoxifen therapy than to screening.)

This finding is very troubling, because we have been made aware of the epidemic of breast cancer by the lay press and the entertainment media and are under the impression that there has been a dramatic rise in the incidence of the disease over the past 25 years. As the incidence of breast cancer has increased, an expensive arsenal of weapons has been brought to bear on the problem, accounting for a cost of $1.2 million spent for each woman benefited by mammography (no one can agree on what "benefited" means).[155] This does not include all the costs of false positive mammograms (something is seen that is insignificant but requires further work-up), legal costs for "missed findings," and emotional costs of detecting cancer that is either so slow growing or nonaggressive as to otherwise have gone unnoticed in the normal life-span of the patient or so aggressive that there is nothing positive that can be done to alter outcome anyway. The adverse physical and psychological effects that accompany false positives are generally underestimated; worry, fearfulness, psychological barriers to appropriate care, stress, pain, and complications from attempts to prove a finding inconsequential are, well, consequential.

The facts are that mortality due to breast cancer has increased by approximately 10 percent since 1970 among women 55 years of age or older and that the recent substantial increase in the use of mammography in women over 50 has not prevented this increase.[118] Among younger women (under 50), the death rate due to breast cancer has declined by almost 25 percent, but the data suggest that declines in mortality were well established before mammography became widely used.[118]

Dr. Plotkin remarks that "the constancy of the death rate in the face of rising incidence and aggressive treatment is a strong hint that we need to approach the disease in another way."[155] He asserts that the increased incidence of breast cancer in American women may well be due to "social progress," in that an enlarging population of intelligent, well-nourished, healthy, productive workforce women are beginning to menstruate earlier (age 12), becoming pregnant later in life and less often, nursing offspring less, and ceasing menses later (age 55) than in the past. They are therefore undergoing 15-20 times the number of menstrual periods as their ancestors. These additional hormonal fluctuations expose the breast tissue to substantially more estrogen/progesterone cycles, which are a major stimulus for cell division, incidents of which can give rise to cancer.[155] These same intelligent women read and think about their health and avail themselves of screening techniques that have been recommended by well-meaning doctors to a much greater degree than did their mothers. Does this mean there is an increased incidence of the disease, or increased awareness, or both?

The behavior of cancer, and its course in patients, is complex and different from infection.

The term "epidemic" properly refers to a disease attacking a large number of people in a population at one time, meaning that lots of individuals are ill or manifesting disease. What is referred to as the "breast cancer epidemic" doesn't really fit the model of an epidemic; mammography is identifying breast cancer in women who have the disorder but are asymptomatic. Breast cancer is not "attacking" the population; we simply have new technology to detect it before it causes symptoms. This seems good at first blush, but following the entire pathway makes the current approach somewhat worrisome.

The confusion around the benefits of screening for breast cancer arises from a leap of logic by physicians and patients who assume that cancer is a disease with a predictable course and a greater probability of cure if detected in early stages. While this reasoning is valid when applied to infectious diseases (for the most part), or to treatment of poisoning for which there is a precise antidote, extrapolation to cancer, given what's know known about tumor behavior, treatment, and cell biology, may be fallacious. Adherence to this model leads the profession and the populace to conclude that early detection effects outcome and suggests that, if doctors look harder and earlier or if patients examine themselves more carefully or take advantage of emerging technology to screen for cancer (PSA levels for prostate cancer, mammograms for breast cancer, stool blood for colon cancer, chest x-rays for lung cancer, etc.), unpleasant outcomes will be avoided.[157,158] This very firmly ingrained idea seems analogous to the tenacious grip physician held to the idea of "miasmas" or "bad humors" as the causes of operative site abscesses, thus negating the truth of infectious microorganisms and the value of washing hands and using antisepsis.

An understanding of the biologic behavior of cancer cells reveals that cancers arising in different tissues vary markedly in their growth characteristics (measured in doubling time) and in their metastatic potential; even tumors arising in the same primary tissue may differ in how aggressively they spread or disseminate on a patient-by-patient basis (prostate and breast cancer are prime examples).

Some tumor types are generally of such low metastatic potential that detection at all, let alone early, has no positive effect on the life-span of patients, because they expire for other reasons.[159] Other tumors (lung, unknown primary adenocarcinoma, and some breast cancers) are so virulent that early diagnosis and therapy have no effect on the outcome. Contrary to conventional thinking, cancers need not attain a critical size in their originating site before spreading, and, conversely, the size of the tumor at the time of diagnosis is often not indicative of metastatic potential.[159]

The behavior of cancer, and its course in patients, is complex and different from infection. Screening, therefore, can be an expensive and invalid way of setting unrealistic expectations in a large number of patients. This is not to say that all screening is inappropriate, and it is certainly not to suggest that methods of detecting pre-neoplastic conditions (such as cervical dysplasia with the pap smear, inspection for dysplastic skin nevi, endoscopy for colon polyps) are unwarranted, but it does suggest that tumors that metastasize before they can be detected and, conversely, those with little metastatic potential regardless of their stage at detection (prostate) are not reasonable candidates for screening.[160]

Breast cancer, which is an amalgam of primary tumors that act unpredictably as far as can be determined by physical examination or mammography, is a classic example of the dilemma. Dr. Plotkin correctly points out that clinicians, patients, and especially lawyers must understand that cancer may be prevented, but it is rarely cured; that it does not progress from small size and low stage to large size prior to spreading distantly in a stepwise fashion; and therefore that early detection, in most cases, is purely incidental with respect to ultimate outcome.[155,160] The fact that we can see or feel the cancer earlier has little to do with what really counts: the aggressiveness and metastatic potential of the tumor just after its first abnormal division and the innately variable ability of each patient's immune system to eradicate the abnormal cells many years before we can detect the cancer by our most sensitive methods.

There is too much confusion and too little information to suggest discontinuing mammography screening, again proving that "cultural authority need not be based on competence—ambiguity may suffice."[161] No time should be wasted collecting comparable data and pursuing research to gain understanding of the entire pathway. Until very recently, there has been no standard for interpreting and reporting mammogram findings. Calcifications, masses, asymmetry, and benign appearances have been freely described according to the ability and judgment of the radiologist. Even now, with standard categorizations by the American College of Radiology, there is nothing to forbid using descriptive terms and phraseology that are noncompliant. Construction of a pathway requires clear comparable data, dedication to looking at costs and benefits of the entire pathway, consideration of ethics in society, and actions consistent with the results of the evidence.

The idea that there is a single "right" way to diagnose or treat illness at lowest possible cost that might be deduced from good capture and analysis of clinical data is simply not a well-ingrained part of the medical tradition.

Dr. Eugene Robin of Stanford has summarized the important elements of any mass screening effort in a healthy population: the screening test should be shown to be accurate and reproducible (insignificant interpretive errors), be subjected to pilot use in a studied subsegment of the population to ensure acceptability, safety, sensitivity (is it missing things), specificity (is it finding things that aren't important or are false positives), and minimal risks of the test to individuals being screened. If the test meets these criteria, it should be applied only in cases where the disease being screened for is an important one for large numbers of people, the problem being detected is acceptably treatable, early detection of the problem leads to demonstrably better outcomes than if it presents later, the disease process is scientifically understood from latency to clinical expression, and the cost of the screening procedure is balanced economically in relation to the benefits of expenditures potentially applicable to other areas of health care.[162]

A complete pathway analysis could also help define when medical miracles are really what they appear to be. Technological miracles have already been mentioned as they apply to intensive care units, but more far reaching analysis suggests enormous expense, unrealistic expectations, and disappointing end product. One example of bleak cardiopulmonary resuscitation results has already been mentioned. In another study, 58 percent of patients were successfully rescued from cardiac arrest, literally "saved." This is a nice step in the pathway. After some incredibly expensive intensive care, however, only 5 percent ever recovered enough to leave the hospital.[163,164] Equally dismal statistics were reported from a 13-year experience at the highly regarded University of Minnesota Bone Marrow Transplant Program, where only three percent of patients who had to be placed on ventilators in ICUs were alive six months later, none who required ventilation within 90 days of transplant lived more than 100 days, and none of the ventilated patients over age 40 lived more than a month.[165] The end product makes one question the means.

PHS has spawned the extremely damaging precept that whatever is done widely in a community; is based on the opinion of experts; or, by virtue of popular use, can be construed as a customary procedure should become a de facto standard of care. This is sometimes referred to as normative validity to distinguish it from scientific validity. The decision that an action is appropriate because of agreements among experts in medicine can be very hazardous; there is almost never widespread agreement among physicians on anything, and the history of normative validity suggests that the process magnifies and perpetuates practices that are ineffective, wasteful, and often wrong.

Such opinion leads to incredible variations in physician practice patterns and to alarming differences in the frequency with which procedures are done for identical conditions (up to a fourfold difference in hysterectomy, tonsillectomy, and prostatectomy within and between states in one study[166]). PHS entitlement explains why 82 different treatment approaches were suggested by 135 family practice doctors for the very common diagnosis of urinary tract infections in women, ranging from very low cost to $250 per case.[167] It similarly accounts for the fact that American general surgery occurs at twice the rate of similar interventions in England, with conservative estimates of more than 3 million unnecessary operations, at a cost of more than $4 billion and directly related deaths of more than 12,000 persons per year.[168]

The same phenomenon explains why, in the United States, 68 percent of heart attack patients need medical imaging studies and 31 percent need surgery, whereas in Canada only 35 percent of myocardial infarction patients need imaging studies and only 12 percent need surgery. The fact that 23 percent of Americans and 22 percent of Canadians died during or soon after treatment leads one to consider the real utility of the studies and the surgery, and it certainly should raise eyebrows to realize that coronary artery bypass surgery in the United States is performed at 10 times the rate it is in Great Britain.[169]

The idea that there is a single "right" way to diagnose or treat illness at lowest possible cost that might be deduced from good capture and analysis of clinical data is simply not a well-ingrained part of the medical tradition; PHS has long propelled Dr. Iatros in the opposite, but sanctified, direction.

A secondary complication of PHS, seen throughout the family lineage, is the trait of inflexibility and difficulty accepting externally imposed or suggested change. This requires no elaboration beyond evidence revealed in the above section on family and developmental history, except to emphasize the fact that information and information technology may well be rejected by Dr. Iatros just as were the enormously beneficial discoveries of Lister, Jenner, Semmelweiss, Laennec, Louis, and a host of others.[170]

Finally, as long as financial gain is linked to number of patients seen or procedures done and the goal of healthy outcomes is disregarded, no amount of information is likely to benefit Dr. Iatros. It is strangely perverse to reward the amount of work done rather than the results of the work, the quality of the work, and the efficiency with which the work was carried out, but this is precisely the case with modern reimbursement and insurance policies.[171] As a result, when good information suggests a change in methods, it appears to be heeded when it indicates more or additional services (and therefore increased remuneration). Because of the perverse way in which care is compensated, new methods, regardless of the nature of supporting evidence, have had a tendency to become additive, as opposed to replacing outmoded methods, and to be overused because they seem safer or less expensive. Evaluations concluding that less should be done are often ignored.[8,45] This is completely opposite to the desirable state, in which the most richly rewarded providers are those who efficiently and rationally learn and navigate treatment pathways to favorable outcomes with minimal resource expenditures.

A unique patient identification number for health records (sometimes called a "master person index") must be legislated and employed on a national basis to enable computerized clinical information to be stored, transmitted, and retrieved accurately by all authorized care providers and health institutions.

New medical technology, patient demands and expectations, and quantity- rather than quality-based remuneration practices clash with economic, ethical, and social imperatives in a most unfortunate way for Dr. Iatros, especially given his personality and the millennia-old tradition of resistance in his culture. Post-Hippocratic syndrome and the conflicts it represents are paralyzing and will require much attention even after the informaciation is cured.

Plan

Orders

Major Depression Treatment

Pharmaceutical treatment for depression in this case, over and above the Prozac Dr. Iatros is currently taking, would only further mask the underlying causes of the condition: Informaciation, Infobia, and Post-Hippocratic Syndrome. Therefore, supportive group therapy is recommended, possibly with oil, bank, airline, or communication industry patients who have had similar problems in the past, while full attention is paid to the root causes of distress.

Grieving work and rebuilding of self-esteem, emphasizing laudable accomplishments, can be worked on, with short-term supportive individual therapy and personal study programs. Because Dr. Iatros does not presently appear to be a danger to himself, suicide precautions seem unnecessary.

Informaciation treatment

A unique patient identification number for health records (sometimes called a "master person index") must be legislated and employed on a national basis to enable computerized clinical information to be stored, transmitted, and retrieved accurately by all authorized care providers and health institutions. A computer-based health record, centered on the patient from birth to death, must facilitate documentation of care grounded in a standardized, common, automatically coded, computer readable medical lexicon.[172] Standard terminology should be used to present alerts and reminders to providers and patients and to support medical decisions with computer logic. It should warn providers of wasteful practices, provide supportive evidence for actions, and present pertinent guidelines for care succinctly and at the moment they are needed.[173,174] It should support and enhance provider decisions with facts about disorders and probabilities of effectiveness to minimize guesswork and mitigate emotional contextual interpretations. Standards for data representation, modeling, and communication must be adhered to regardless of application interfaces and sites or settings of care.

Standard terminology should be used to present alerts and reminders to providers and patients and to support medical decisions with computer logic. It should warn providers of wasteful practices, provide supportive evidence for actions, and present pertinent guidelines for care succinctly and at the moment they are needed.

The computer-based health record must be designed in conjunction with health care providers to match collection and communication of concise, relevant, comparable, clinically accurate patient information with efficient care delivery processes. The record must make information available to multiple users simultaneously and in geographically dispersed locales, and network infrastructure should be leveraged or created to support high-bandwidth data and image transfer capacity for purposes of remote medical consultation and treatment along with care documentation. It must be available to a full spectrum of health care providers, easily handed off from provider to provider on teams, and designed to support the shift in clinical responsibilities from physicians to medical assistants, nurses, and, ultimately, patients.

Demonstrate that information can be used positively to enhance the health and vitality of patients, the satisfaction of clinicians, and the human relationship elements of the care process.

Patient data in the computerized health record must be secure and transmitted with sufficient encryption to ensure appropriate confidentiality and must be presented to users in a familiar, intuitive clinical context. It must present an integrated user interface, such that provider actions and documentation need be done only once and can subsequently be displayed wherever appropriate without duplication of effort. The interface should also support the mind-mapping nature of clinical thought processes, optimize information availability without compromising completeness, and improve efficiency for the clinician.

Programs should be established with employers, insurers, and patients to reward clinicians for use of the computer-based health record; for compliance with established clinical guideline; for shifts from wasteful practices to more effective disease prevention, health promotion, and patient education activities based on scientific evidence; and for shifts from today's "more equals quality" methods.[174,175]

National and health organization-specific data warehouses should be established and be based on a common lexicon and data model to allow for valid information comparisons and migration between databases regardless of which proprietary medical record application might be used to document care. Clinical information should be analyzed to gain understanding of effective medical interventions and to predict areas in which health can be proactively maintained rather than repaired. The new information system must be built with the capacity to change and evolve with expanding knowledge of best processes, such that alerts, reminders, guidelines, and logic are flexible and modifiable in the context of rapid changes.

Infobia Orders

Tailor technology introduction, system design and training, user education, and post-implementation support to the idiosyncrasies of the medical culture, understanding the genesis of fears surrounding the changes to be instituted. Prepare clinicians with the technical, historical, and philosophical background needed for movement into the information age before introducing technology, understanding that, just as with the use of the stethoscope or the vaginal speculum, more rapid progress will be made if the system is "warmed before use" and the patient is prepared for the contact. Recognize the faces and the manifestations of infobia, including fears of loss of autonomy, improper outside controls, and diminished care quality and address them head on, with honesty and integrity. Demonstrate that information can be used positively to enhance the health and vitality of patients, the satisfaction of clinicians, and the human relationship elements of the care process. Emphasize that resistance to information systems will compel less educated and more ill-motivated outsiders to control activities on the basis of economics and emotion rather than of medical science.

Post-Hippocratic Syndrome Orders

Insist on a shift in medical education processes to teach acceptance of information systems as enhancements to care. De-emphasize brutal tactics in the education of physicians and the resultant reflexive antagonistic resistance to change. Select candidates for medical education based on reasoning ability, compassion, flexibility, understanding of ethics, and healthy attitudes toward family and humanity, as opposed to memorization capacity, scholastic performance, and irrelevant academic test scores. Make students more aware of their own limitations as well as those of medical knowledge and teach them the importance of pathway analysis and balanced skepticism in evaluation and use of new technology, as well as the crucial role of human behavior in health and health care.[2,163] Imbue them with respect for the iatrogenic potential of their interventions, and emphasize listening to their patients and advising them on health matters with scientific wisdom and human compassion.

Eliminate habitual use of medical diagnostic tools and technology, including unproved screening procedures; curtail use of advanced modalities for imaging; eschew new methods of chemical analysis; avoid emerging invasive or surgical techniques; and prescribe no new medicines unless there is clear scientific evidence of both immediate and long-term benefit from such interventions. (Given that the sevenfold increase in health care spending since 1950 is largely due to new technology and additive practice patterns, an appropriateness filter on technology use could predictably result in savings estimated at between $50 and $200 billion per year without a deleterious effect on health.) Use established diagnostic and treatment technology only when the information that will result from its application will have a significant effect on choices of treatment, and apply tests and treatments only in the context of definite benefits. Dubious medical technology is particularly dangerous because it actually further reduces clinical autonomy by making caregivers subject to control by whoever supplies the capital for the equipment.[177]

Clinicians must be conditioned to ask questions in every instance and at every decision point. Is this necessary? Will it alter my treatment? Is it proved? Is it accurate and reliable? Am I taking action to protect me legally or to contribute to improved health in my patient? Do the patient and I understand the risks, costs, and benefits of the action? If the patient and I were to directly share the expenses and the

Work to facilitate a shift of fiscal responsibility from insurers and employers to health care providers and patients; enlist support from other professionals for changes needed in legal and legislative arenas; and act responsibly and respectably in the best interests of patients collectively, recognizing and teaching the benefits of this approach to them.

consequences of the action, would I recommend it and would he or she pursue it? Identical questions must be asked of care providers by patients in an insistent and persistent way, which is more likely to occur if there are direct financial consequences for involved parties in the mutual interrogation.

Directly involve patients in responsibility for their health care decisions, including financial responsibility for noncompliance or unhealthy life-styles. Using education and financial incentives, shift patient expectations of care into a pattern consistent with evidence and analysis and away from maximalist expectations and entitlement. Develop the basis and the courage to say "no" to patients, patients' families, and legislators when treatments or interventions are not in the best interests of patients or do not support their function as human beings who can carry on life with dignity.[178] Work to facilitate a shift of fiscal responsibility from insurers and employers to health care providers and patients; enlist support from other professionals for changes needed in legal and legislative arenas; and act responsibly and respectably in the best interests of patients collectively, recognizing and teaching the benefits of this approach to them. Provide strong support for patients in addressing preventable causes of illness and injury generally viewed as social ills (tobacco, drugs, violence).[43]

Disposition

Dr. Iatros is approaching a premorbid state and will rapidly enter a futile care state without appropriate intervention. Only he can alter his course and begin self-regulation and recovery.[179] Unfortunately, information system therapy is costly but essential; without it, measurement and precise comparisons of treatments, risks, benefits, and outcomes across the patient population cannot be done. (This is not to say that all things can be measured, but by now one should be able to see that there is considerable room for improvement.) There is enough waste within the current system to pay for the infrastructure necessary to allow discovery of more effective ways of practicing, but it is unclear if Dr. Iatros has the strength and capability to change rapidly enough to use it to survive.

Prognosis remains guarded, because, even if recommended informaciation therapy is carried out, actualization of gains from the treatment still depend on far reaching changes in medical culture.[180] As determinations of what constitutes effective care emerge, financial incentives to change clinician behavior in the right direction, along with protection from irrational legal and legislative reprisals for taking proper actions, will have to be formulated.[181] Public support will need to be garnered for a migration to principled methods of evidence-based practice in which no test, procedure, or treatment is undertaken for which there is no demonstrable proof of benefit.

Dr. Iatros can recover if he begins to see himself as an entity consisting of interconnected parts, each requiring energy and using resources in the process of diagnosing and treating illness. Because these aggregate parts influence each other, they must interact in a balanced way for the entire structure to survive. A transition from dispersed, isolated, self-sustaining, fee-for-service medical cost centers, each acting in a unicellular fashion and seeking to maximize individual viability, to a more cooperative "animal" coordinated by information communication and feedback will need to evolve. Absent such cooperation, the American approach to medicine will continue to be, as Halvorson decries, "a nonsystem with no accountability for care outcomes, no tracking of performance, and no financial incentive to work together to create and standardize best practices and care protocols."[182]

Care team coordination, communication, specialization, and integration through information systems will enable balanced efficiency and allow the system to focus on overall quality and value. This balance will require comfort among providers about their precise responsibilities and about their pivotal roles in society as a whole.[183]

A key element of this living fabric is the patient, healthy or ill. Dr. Iatros must insist that his patients participate in health decisions, act as informed consumers, and bear more direct moral and financial responsibility for cooperative decisions. Physician and author Melvin Konner accurately observed that "Few patients understand how many decisions are a toss up, and how bleak and forbidding the landscape of disease can look even to those who know more about it than anyone else in the world. Doctors, scientists, and journalists have given us all—including themselves—such a hard sell about advances in medicine that only the most sophisticated ever go to a physician any more without overestimating what the physician can do."[184] This is one of the highest risks to Dr. Iatros' recovery, because, as eminent surgeon Dr. Denton Cooley has observed: "Americans believe that health is a state of perfection....Our society's preoccupation with beauty has made our plastic surgeons rich and our young girls sick with eating disorders. Length of life has become more important than quality of life. Consequently, the lives of terminally ill patients are extended by ventilators or other measures of extraordinary care. Our society lives in denial of death, as if, with enough knowledge and technology, it were possible to stave it off somehow."[185]

If the simple criterion of appropriateness, based on accurate evidence, is applied with compassion, confidence, and wisdom, dramatic improvement in Dr. Iatros' condition is possible. Recovery will likely be prolonged, as healing will not begin until debridement is completed, toxic data are expunged, standards are accepted, and balance is attained, perhaps for the first time in history.

Only through knowledge and the demonstration of effective clinical methods can the economic relationship between insurance, government, and health care providers be favorably altered such that medicine is returned to the hands of caregivers and care receivers, where everything began. Dr. Iatros' mission after recovery will no longer be to exclude every obscure diagnosis in each patient, disregarding odds and cost, but rather to discover, improve, and promulgate techniques for maintaining health and achieving the best disease management outcomes over a fair distribution of society.

In attempting to arrive at the truth, I have applied everywhere for information, but in scarcely an instance have I been able to obtain hospital records for any purposes of comparison. If they could be obtained, they would enable us to decide many questions besides the one alluded to. They would show subscribers how their money was being spent, what amount of good was really being done with it, and whether the money was doing mischief rather than good.— Florence Nightingale, American Nurse, 1873

References

1. Illich, I. *Medical Nemesis*. New York, N.Y.: Pantheon, 1976, p. 41.
2. Mendelsohn, R. *Confessions of a Medical Heretic*. Chicago, Ill.: Contemporary Books, 1979.
3. Kilbourne, P. "Public Growing Colder Toward Managed Care, Polls find." *Denver Post*, Sept.28,1997, p.11a.
4. Tenner, E. *Why Things Bite Back: Technology and the Revenge of Unintended Consequences*. New York, N.Y.: Knopf, 1996, p. 34.
5. Conklin, M. "Doctors in Distress." *Rocky Mountain News*, Dec. 15, 1996, p. lb.
6. Stolberg, S. "As Patients Learn, Doctors Worry." *Rocky Mountain News*, Sept. 9, 1997, p.60.
7. Konner, M. *Medicine at the Crossroads*. New York, N.Y.: Vintage Books, 1994, p.256.
8. Eddy, D. "Three Battles to Watch in the 1990s." *JAMA* 270(4):520-6, July 28, 1993.
9. Halvorson, G., *Strong Medcine*, New York, N.Y.: Random House, p.49.
10. Eddy, D., and Billings, S. "The Quality of Medical Evidence: Implications for Quality of Care." *HealthAffairs* 7(1):19-32, Spring 1988.
11. Dixon, B. *Beyond the Magic Bullet*. New York, N.Y.: Harper and Row, 1978, p. 3.
12. Rollman, B., and others. "Medical Specialty and the Incidence of Divorce." *New England Journal of Medicine* 336(11):800-3, March 13, 1997.
13. Roy, A. "Suicide in Doctors." *Psychiatric Clinics of North America* 8(2):377-87, June 1985.
14. Majno, G. *The Healing Hand: Man and Wound in the Ancient World*. Cambridge, Mass; Harvard Universoity Press, 1991.

15.   Ghalioungli, P. *Magic and Medical Science in Ancient Egypt.* London, Endland: Hoddon and Stoughton, 1963.

16.   Majno, G., *op. cit.*, pp. 229-260

17.   Cartwright, F., and Biddiss, M. *Disease and History.* New York, N.Y.: Barnes and Noble Books, 1972, p.20.

18.   Gordon, R. *The Alarming History of Medicine.* New York, N.Y.: St. Martins Press, 1993, p.6.

19.   Cartwright, F., and Biddiss, M., *op.cit.*, p.24

20.   Gordon, R., *op. cit.*, p.56.

21.   Cartwright, F., and Biddiss, M. op.cit., pp. 82-112.

22.   McGrew, R. *Encyclopedia of Medical History.* New York, N.Y.: McGraw-Hill Book Company, 1985, p. 69.

23.   Boswell, J. *Life of Samuel Johnson*, L.F. Powell's revision of G. B. Hill's edition, Vol. 1, p. 91n, from reviews of Dr. Lucas's "Essay on Waters", Nov. 25, 1734.

24.   Lyons, A., and Petrucelli, R. Medicine: *An Illustrated History.* New York, N.Y.: Harry N. Abrams, Inc., 1978, p. 513.

25.   Gordon, R., *op. cit.*, p. 170.

26.   Starr, P. *The Transformation of American Medicine.* Harper Collins Publishers, 1982, p. 42.

27.   Gordon, R. An *Alarming History of Famous and Difficult Patients.* New York, N.Y.: St. Martin's Press, 1997, pp. 29-31.

28.   Tenner, E., *op. cit.*, p. 32.

29.   Schneiderman, L., and Jecker, N. *Wrong Medicine: Doctors, Patients, and Futile Treatment.* Baltimore, Md.: Johns Hopkins University Press, 1995.

30.   James, A. *"Ethics in Current Medical Imaging."* American Journal of Roentgenology 160(1):1-4, Jan. 1993.

31.   Starr, P., *op cit.*, p. 136.

32.   McGrew, R., *op. cit.*, p. 75.

33.   Starr, P., *op cit.*, pp. 134-44.

34.   Herman, P., and others. "Disagreements in Chest Roentgen Interpretation." *Chest* 68(3):278-82, Sept. 1975.

35.   Halvorson, G., *op. cit.*, p. 16.

36.   Hillman, B., and others. "Frequency and Costs of Diagnostic Imaging in Office Practice." *New England Journal of Medicine* 323(23):1604-8, Dec. 6, 1990

37.   Hillman, B., and others. "Physician Utilization and Charges for Outpatient Diagnostic Imaging in a Medicare Population." *JAMA* 268(15):2050-4, Oct. 21, 1992.

38.   Swedlow, A., and others. "Increased Costs and Rates of Use in the California Workers' Compensation System as a Result of Self-Referral by Physicians." *New England Journal of Medicine* 327(21):1502-6, Nov. 19, 1992.

39.   Reynolds, R., and others. "The Costs of Medical Professional Liability." *JAMA* 257(20):2776-81, May 22, 1987.

40.   Schneiderman, L., and Jecker, N., *op. cit.*, p.85.

41.   Rifkin, J. *Entropy.* New York, N.Y.: Bantam Books, 1980, p. 274.

42.   Pelke, S., and others. "Gowning Does Not Affect Colonization or Infection Rates in a Neonatal Intensive Care Unit." *Archives of Pediatric and Adolescent Medicine* 148(10):1016-20, Oct. 1994.

43.   Berwick, D. "Run to Space: Plenary Address to the National Institute for Healthcare Improvement, 7th Annual National Forum of Quality Improvement in Healthcare, Dec. 6, 1995.

44.   Elliott, G. "Computer-Assisted Quality Assurance: Development and Performance of a Respiratory Care Program." *Quality Review Bulletin* 17(3):85-90, Mar. 1991.

45.   Berwick, D. "Eleven Worthy Aims for Clinical Leadership in Health System Reform." *JAMA* 272(10):797-802, Sept. 14, 1994.

46.   Field, S., and others. "The Erect Abdominal Film of the Acute Abdomen: Should Its Routine Use Be Abandoned?" *British Medical Journal* 290(6486):1934-6, June 29, 1985.

47.   Mirvis, S. "Plain Film Evaluation of Patients with Abdominal Pain: Are Three Radiographs Necessary?" *American Journal of Roentgenology* 147(3):501-3, Sept. 1986.

48.   Ewigman, B., and others. "Effect of Ultrasound Screening on Perinatal Outcome." *New England Journal of Medicine* 329(12):821-7, Sept. 1993.

49.   Hall, F. "Overutilization of Radiologic Examinations." *Radiology* 120(2):443-8, Aug. 1976.

50.   Thornbury, J., and others. "Hypertensive Urogram: A Nondiscriminatory Test for Renovascular Hypertension." *American Journal of Roentgenology* 138(1):43-9, Jan. 1982.

51.   Masters, S., and others. "Skull X-Ray Examinations after Trauma; Recommendations by a Multidisciplinary Panel and Validation Study. *New England Journal of Medicine* 316(2):84-91, Jan. 8, 1987.

52.   Robin, E. *Matters of Life and Death: Risks vs. Benefits of Medical Care.* Palo Alto, Calif.: Stanford Alumni Association, 1984.

53.   Narr, B. "Outcomes of Patients with No Laboratory Assessment before Anesthesia and a Surgical Procedure." *Mayo Clinic Proceedings* 72:505-9, 1997.

54.   Starr, P., *op.cit.* p. 30-3.

55.   *Ibid.*, pp. 88-106.

56.   *Ibid.*, p. 113.

57.   Lyons, A., *op. cit.*, p. 534.

58.   Starr. P., *op. cit.* p. 137.

59.   Rifkin, J., *op. cit.*, p. 175.

60.   Eddy, D. "What Do We Do about Costs?" *JAMA* 254(9):1161-70, Sept. 5, 1990.

61.   Thorpe, K. "Health Care Cost Containment." In Kovner, A., Editor, *Jonas's Health Care Delivery in the United States.* New York, N.Y.: Springer, 1994, p. 295.

62.   Reagan, M. *Curing the Crisis: Options for American's Health Care.* Boulder, Colorado: Westview Press, 1992, p.50

63.   Broder, D. "Health Care Crisis Is Back." *Denver Post* "Perspectives," p. I-3, Oct. 26, 1991.

64.   *Ibid.*, p.14

65.   Easterbrook, G. "The Revolution." *Newsweek*, Jan 26, 1987, p. 74.

66.   Konner, M., op. cit., pp. xiii-xxvii

67.   Blendon, R. "Three Systems: A Comparative Survey." *Health Management Quarterly* 11(1):2, 1989.

68. Analysis released April 26, 1996, American College of Physicians, Philadelphia, Pa., and Williamson, B. "Malpractice Suits Drive Up the Cost of Health Care." *International Journal of Issues in Medicine*, Dec. 1995.
69. Broder, D., *op. cit.*
70. Schneiderman, L. and Jecker, N., *op. cit.*, pp. 8-13.
71. Kovner, A. "Introduction." In Kovner, A., Editor, *Jonas's Health Care Delivery in the United States*. New York, N.Y.: Springer, 1994, p. 5.
72. Starfield, B. *Primary Care: Concept, Evaluation, and Policy*. New York, N.Y.: Oxford University Press, 1992.
73. Reagan, M., *op.cit.*, pp. 6,53.
74. Halvorson, G., *op. cit.*, p. 3.
75. Meadow, W. University of Chicago Survey reported in *Pediatrics Electronic Pages*, May 1997.
76. Miller, C. "Infant Mortality in the United States." *Scientific American* 253(1):31-7, July 1985.
77. Chiles, L. "National Commission to Prevent Child Mortality." *Mothering*, Summer 1988, p. 67.
78. Lake, J. "Prenatal Care: A Cost-Effective Approach." *Journal of Advances in Child Care*, July 1995.
79. McDuffy, R., and others. "The Effect of Frequency of Prenatal Care Visits on Perinatal Outcome Among Low-Risk Women: A Randomized Controlled Trial." *JAMA* 275(11):847-51, March 20, 1996.
80. Banta, H. "Health Care and Health Reform." In Kovner, A., Editor, *Jonas's, Health Care Delivery in the United States*. New York, N.Y.: Springer, 1994, p. 28.
81. Robin, E., *op. cit.*, p. 102.
82. Schneiderman, L., and Jecker, N., *op cit.*, pp.45,71.
83. Blackhall, W. "Must We Always Use CPR?" *New England Journal of Medicine* 317(20):1281-5, Nov.12, 1987.
84. Dixon, B., *op. cit.*, p. 226.
85. Brook, R., and Lohr, K. "Will We Need to Ration Effective Health Care? *Issues in Science and Technology* 3:1-10, 1986.
86. Rifkin, J., *op. cit.*, p. 176.
87. Van Bemmel, *op. cit.*, p. 8
88. Thorpe, K., *op. cit.*, p. 294.
89. Halvorson, G., *op. cit.*, p. 83.
90. Konner, M., *op. cit.*, p. 86.
91. *Ibid.*, p. 84.
92. *Harvard Heart Letter*, Dec. 2, 1991, p. 8.
93. Berman, S., and others." Otitis Media-Related Antibiotic Prescribing Patterns, Outcomes, and Expenditures in a Pediatric Medicaid Population." *Pediatrics* 100(4):585-92, Oct.1997.
94. Molotsky, I. "Animal Antibiotics Tied to Illnesses in Humans." *New York Times*, Feb. 22, 1987.
95. Fisher, J. *The Plague Makers*. New York, N.Y.: Simon and Schuster, 1994, p. 31.
96. Gonzales, R., and others. "Antibiotic Prescribing for Adults with Colds, Upper Respiratory Tract Infections, and Bronchitis by Ambulatory Care Physicians." *JAMA* 278(11):901-4, Sept. 17, 1997.
97. Rifkin, J., *op. cit.*, p. 177.

98.   Silverman, M., and Lee, P. *Pills, Profits, and Politics*. Berkeley, Calif.: University of California Press, 1974.

99.   Johannes, L., and Strecklow, S. "Diet Pill Sales Plummet as Medical Concerns Rise." *Wall Sreet Jounral*, Sept. 4, 1997.

100.   Cartwright, I. and Biddiss, M. *op. cit.*, pp. 215-8.

101.   Brennan, T., and others. "Incidence of Adverse Effects and Negligence in Hospitalized Patients: Results of the Harvard Medical Practice Study, Part 1." *New England Journal of Medicine* 324(6):370-6, Feb. 7, 1991.

102.   Leape, L. "The Nature of Adverse Events in Hospitalized Patients: Results of the Harvard Medical Practice Study, Part 2." *New England Journal of Medicine* 324(6):377-84, Feb. 7, 1991.

103.   Tenner, E., *op. cit.*, p. 42.

104.   Office of Technology Assessment. "Assessing the Efficacy and Safety of Medical Technologies." Pub. No. OTA-H-75, 1978a. Washington, D.C.: U.S. Government Printing Office, 1978.

105.   Aaron, H., and Schwartz, W. *The Painful Prescription: Rationing Hospital Care*. Washington, D.C.: The Brooking Institution, 1984.

106.   Banta, H., and Thacker, S. "Assessing the Costs and Benefits of Routine Fetal Monitoring." *Obstetric and Gynecologic Survey* 34(8):627-42, Aug. 1979.

107.   Kosecoff, J., and others. "Obtaining Clinical Data on the Appropriateness of Medical Care in Community Practice." *JAMA* 258(18):2538-42, Nov. 13, 1987.

108.   Banta, D., and Kemp, K. *Management of Health Care Technology in 9 Countries*. New York, N.Y.: Springer, 1982.

109.   Leutwyler, K. "The Price of Prevention." *Scientific American* 272(4):124-9, April 1995.

110.   Tenner, E., *op. cit.*, p. 28.

111.   Rifkin, J., *op. cit.*, p. 178.

112.   McKeown, T. *The Role of Medicine, Dream, Mirage, or Nemesis*. Oxford, England: Basil and Blackwell, 1979.

113.   Robin, E., *op. cit.*, p. 41.

114.   Tenner, E., *op. cit.*, p. 30.

115.   Banta, H., and Jonas, S. "Health and Health Care." In Kovner, A., Editor, *Jonas's Health Care Delivery in the United States*. New York, N.Y.: Springer, 1994, p. 18.

116.   Kovner, A., *op. cit.*, p. 4.

117.   "Select Cancer Facts," http://kci.wayne.edu:80/facts html, Jan. 8, 1997.

118.   Bailar, J., and Gornick, H. "Cancer Undefeated." *New England Journal of Medicine* 336(22):1569-74, May 29, 1997.

119.   Parker, S., and others. "Cancer Incidence, Survival, and Mortality Data." *CA: Cancer Journal for Clinicians* 46(1):5-27, Jan.-Feb. 1996.

120.   Schneiderman, L., and Jecker, N., *op. cit.*, pp. 24-5.

121.   Robin, E., *op. cit.*, p. 47.

122.   Starr. P., *op. cit.*, p. 5.

123.   Banta, H., and Jonas, S., *op. cit.*, p 26.

124.   Weitzman, B. "Improving Quality of Care." In Kovner, A., Editor, *Jonas's, Health Care Delivery in the United States*. New York, N.Y.: Springer, 1994, p. 378.

125.   Dick, R., and Steen, E., Editors. *The Computer-Based Patient Record*. Washington, D.C.: National Academy Press, 1991, p. 15.

126. Gabrielli, E. "Electronic Ambulatory Medical Record." *Journal of Clinical Computing* 28(2):27-53, 1989.
127. Dick, R., *op. cit.*, p. 17.
128. Weed, L. "The Problem-Oriented Record as a Basic Tool in Medical Education, Patient Care, and Research." *Annals of Clinical Research* 3(3):131-4, June 1971.
129. Humphries, B., and others, "Evaluating the Coverage of Controlled Health Data Terminologies: Report on the Results of the NLM/AHCPR Large-Scale Vocabulary Test." *Journal of the American Medical Informatics Association* 4(6):484-500, Nov.-Dec. 1997.
130. Von Bemmel, *op. cit.*, pp. 80-98.
131. Chute, C., and others. "Multi-Institutional Test Bed for C l i n i c a l Vocabulary: Grant Application to U.S. Department of Health and Human Services, April 26, 1994.
132. Tierney, W., and others. "The Effect on Test Ordering of Informing Physicians of the Charges for Outpatient Diagnostic Tests." *New England Journal of Medicine* 322(21):1499-504, May 24, 1990.
133. Tierney, W., and others. "Computer Predictions of Abnormal Test Results: Effects on Outpatient Testing." *JAMA* 259(8):1194-8, Feb. 26, 1988.
134. Tierney, W., and others. "Physician Inpatient Order Writing on Microcomputer Workstations: Effects on Resource Utilization." *JAMA* 269(3):379-83, Jan 20, 1993.
135. Shea, S., and others. "Computer General Informational Messages Directed to Physicians: Effect on Length of Hospital Stay." *Journal of the American Medical Informatics Association* 2(1):58-64, Jan.-Feb. 1995.
136. Schriger, D., and others "Implementation of Clinical Guidelines Using a Computer Charting System." *JAMA* 278(19):, 585-90, Nov. 19, 1987.
137. Chute, C., and others. "The Content Coverage of Clinical Classifications." *Journal of the American Medical Informatics Association* 3(3):224-31, May-June 1996.
138. Halvorson, G., *op. cit.*, pp. 25-7.
139. Mongerson, P. "A Patient's Perspective of Medical Informatics." *Journal of the American Medical Informatics Association* 2(2):79-84, March-April 1995.
140. Reagan, D., *op. cit.*, p. 130
141. Attendorf, A., and Attendorf, T. *ISMs: A Compendium of Concepts, Doctrines, Traits, and Beliefs.* Memphis, Tenn., Mustang Publishing Co., 1993.
142. Tenner, E., *op. cit.*, p. 41.
143. *Ibid.*, p. 43.
144. Banta, H. "Technology Assessment in Health Care." In Kovner, A., Editor, *Jonas's, Health Care Delivery in the United States.* New York, N.Y.: Springer, 1994, p. 415.
145. Schneiderman, L., and Jecker, N., op. cit., p. 44
146. Gurney, J. "Why Chest Radiography Became Routine." *R a d i o l o g y* 195(1):245-6, April 1995.
147. Osler, W. *The Principles and Practice of Medicine.* Edinburgh, Scotland: Young and Pentland, 1898.
148. Garland, L. "Studies on the Accuracy of Diagnostic Procedures." *American Journal of Roentgenology* 82(1):25-38, Jan. 1959.

149. Berlin, L. "Does the 'Missed' Radiographic Diagnosis Constitute Malpractice?" *Radiology* 123(2):523-7, May 1977.
150. Whalen, J., and Balter, S. *Radiation Risks in Medical Imaging.* Chicago, Ill.: Yearbook Medical Publishers, 1984.
151. Tape, T., and Mushlin, A. "How Useful Are Routine Chest X-Rays of Preoperative Patients at Risk for Postoperative Chest Disease?" *Journal of General Internal Medicine* 3(1):15-20, Jan.-Feb. 1988.
152. Fowkes, F. "The Value of Routine Preoperative Chest X-Rays."*British Journal of Hospital Medicine* 35(2):120-3, Feb. 1986.
153. Eddy, D. "'Screening for Lung Cancer." *Annals of Internal Medicine* 111(3):232-7, April 1989.
154. Gurney, J., *op. cit.*, p. 246.
155. Plotkin, D. "The Good News and the Bad News about Breast Cancer." *Atlantic Monthly*, June 1996, p. 76.
156. National Cancer Institute Cancer Web, http://www.graylab. ac.uk.8080/cancernet/ 600625.html, Jan. 8, 1997.
157. Jacobson, P. "Medical Malpractice and the Tort System." *JAMA* 262(23):3320-7, Dec. 15, 1981.
158. Robin, E., *op. cit.*, p. 133.
159. Meyers, F. "Screening for Cancer: Is It Worth It?" *Western Journal of Medicine* 163(2):166-8, Aug. 1995.
160. Meyers, F. "Tumor Biology in Explanation of Failure of Screening for Cancer and in Determining Future Strategies." *American Journal of Medicine* 80(5):911-6, May 1986.
161. Starr, P., *op. cit.* p. 140.
162. Robin, E., *op. cit.*, pp. 122-3.
163. Halvorson, G., *op. cit.*, p. 93.
164. "Cost of Heart Revival Found to be $150,000 per Survivor." *Wall Street Journal*, March 21, 1993, p. 15.
165. Schneiderman, L., and Jecker, N., *op. cit.*, p. 46
166. Wennberg, J. "Dealing with Medical Practice Variations: A Proposal for Action." *Health Affairs* 3(2):6-32, Summer 1984.
167. Berg, A. "Variations among Family Physicians: Management Strategies for Lower Urinary Tract Infections in Women. A Report from the Washington Family Physician Collaborative Research Network." *Journal of the American Board of Family Practice* 4(5):327-30, Sept.-Oct. 1991.
168. McPherson, K. "International Differences in Medical Care Practices." *Health Care Financing Review,* Annual Supplement, 1989, pp. 6-20.
169. Rouleau, J., and others. "A Comparison of Management Patterns after Acute Myocardial Infarction in Canada and the United States." *New England Journal of Medicine* 328(11):779-84, March 18, 1993.
170. Robin, E., *op. cit.*, p. 67.
171. Reagan, D., *op. cit.*, p. 67.
172. Spackman, K., and others,"A Reference Terminology for Health Care." *Proceedings of AMIA, A Fall Symposium*, Oct. 1997. Philadelphia, Pa.: Hanley and Belfus, Inc., pp. 640-4.
173. Eddy, D. A *Manual for Assessing Health Practices and Designing Practice Policies: The Explicit Approach.* Philadelphia, Pa: American College of Physicians, 1992.
174. Cohn, S., and Chute, C. "Clinical Terminology and Computer-Based Patient Records." *JAMIA* 68(2):41-3, Feb. 1997.

175. Bree, R., and others. "Effect of Mandatory Radiology Consultation on Inpatient Imaging Use; A Randomized Controlled Trial." *JAMA* 276(19):1595-8, Nov. 20, 1996.

176. Pearson, S., and others. "Critical Pathways as a Strategy for Improving Care: Problems and Potential." *Annals of Internal Medicine* 123 (12):941-8, Dec. 15, 1995.

177. Starr, P., *op. cit.*, p. 16.

178. Schneiderman, L., and Jecker, N., *op. cit.*, pp. 60, 88.

179. Robin, E., *op. cit.*, pp. 179-80.

180. Harpole, L., and others."Automated Evidence—Based Critiquing of Orders for Abdominal Radiographs: Impacts on Utilization and Appropriateness. *Journal of American Medical Informatics.* 4(6):511-21, Nov.-Dec. 1997.

181. Ellrodt, G., and others. "Evidence-Based Disease Management." *JAMA* 278(20):1687-91, Nov. 26, 1997.

182. Halvorson, G., *op. cit.*, p. 56.

183. Eddy, D. "Broadening the Responsibility of Practitioners: The Team Approach." *JAMA* 269(14):1849-55, April 14, 1993.

184. Konner, M., *op. cit.*, p.25.

185. Cooley, D. "Medical Practice: Past, Present, Future." *The Pharos* 60(1):13-6, Winter 1997.

Information System Basics

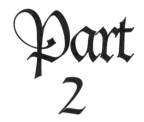

Part 2

The chapters in this part of the book introduce the language and concepts any computer user needs as a base from which to expand his or her understanding of the information age, regardless of profession. Health care workers with no knowledge of information systems may find the new terminology a little imposing at first, so I encourage them to look for humor as they read as anchors for the fresh knowledge.

Those with intermediate to expert knowledge of computers and systems may see familiar terms in a new light and may be able to use the revealed ironies and insights to teach others their language more effectively. Amusement is a very helpful medium for bridging cultures, alleviating tension, and ameliorating fear.

If an area seems too arcane, skim it and move on; even cursory knowledge will be enough to get started, and one can always come back later. Words that are italicized are further defined in the book's lexicon

In a time of drastic change, it is the learners who inherit the future. The learned usually find themselves equipped to live in a world that no longer exists.—Eric Hoffer, U.S. philosopher, longshoreman, 1973.

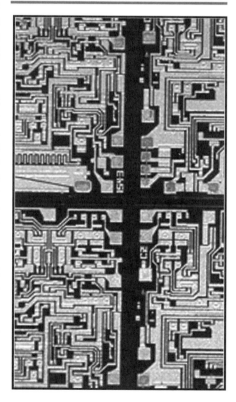

Chapter 2

COMPUTER HARDWARE

Other creatures must rely on their own anatomy—their eyes, ears, nose, teeth, claws, and so on—to gather energy. Human beings, however, because of our more highly developed nervous system and brain, have succeeded in augmenting and extending our natural biological apparatus with the creation of all sorts of tools.—Jeremy Rifkin, American economist and activist, 1980.

The elements of a computer information system that can be broken with a hammer are *hardware*. For all practical purposes, hardware consists of *computers* and their essential physical innards and *peripheral devices* that augment the functions of the computer.

Computers

Computers are machines that accept data input, process that data in a defined manner, and present the results of processing in a fashion that is comprehensible to the user. The essential hardware component of a modern computer is its central processing unit (CPU), which consists of silicon microprocessors called "chips" and micro-electronic pathways.

The energy that circulates within and between the hardware devices is predominantly electrical. This energy can induce changes in arrays of infinitesimal switches on the chips, depending on whether the electrical message makes a positive or a negative impression. The aggregated sequence of positive and negative impressions amount to data. (If you work in a large organization you may wish to compare this to your position in the company, which similarly depends on a series of positive or negative impressions on others, the aggregate of which is a career move.)

Bits

Recognize that all of the activities in computing can be reduced to the fact that tiny micro-switches are in a positive or a negative state (on or off). Because there are only two possible impressions that the electrical energy can induce for each switch, the basis of computing is referred to as "binary" (two by two), and because these two states are represented by "digits," 0 for off and 1 for on, the smallest unit that can be represented is called a binary digit—a bit. When energy has been transformed into binary digits for use by computers, it is said to have been made digital. Information, therefore, is just filtered or connected data, which you now understand can always be blown to bits.

It is not important to understand exactly how computers create and store data or massage it into information, but, just as one cannot intelligently discuss finance without understanding the core currency, one cannot wax eloquent about information systems without being familiar with the bit.

Bytes

It takes a number of bits to represent, or "encode," a single character of data on the chip. This package of bits is called a byte. The byte is the entity moved as a single unit by a particular microprocessor. Different chips can handle different sized bit packages as byte units. You will hear people talk about "32-bit" or "64-bit" systems.

When energy has been transformed into binary digits for use by computers, it is said to have been made digital.

It is now time to introduce Rose's acronym, which can be applied to virtually all elements of computing: BOFIB (bigger or faster is better). One wants a 64-bit system, unless something bigger comes along, particularly if the system is for you personally.

Kilo, Mega, Giga, Tera

BOFIB requires a discussion of measurement and comparison. Bits are packaged into bytes, and a single byte encodes one character of data. Visualize a byte as a single note on a page of a Beethoven symphonic musical score. (Remember, this is not a book for dummies.)

In the metric system, a thousand of something is a "kilo." A page of the symphonic score contains about a kilobyte (1,000 bytes) of notes. A thousand kilobytes are called a "megabyte," which is therefore a million bytes total. A thousand megabytes is called a "gigabyte" (a billion bytes), and a thousand gigabytes is a "terabyte" (way too many zeros).

Floppy disk storage and random access memory (RAM) are measured in megabytes, whereas hard disk and compact disc storage is measured in gigabytes. You don't want to clutter your mind with the notion of the paltry kilobyte from here on.

Boards

Chips and micro-electronics are fastened to or embedded in a fiberglass "board" also called a "card." The central processing unit card is called the motherboard or "logic board." In the past, these boards were given class numbers and letter designations such as 386DX or 486SX, but, since the introduction of the new Pentium® chip by Intel Corporation, they have been identified by the speed with which they can process transactions. The speed is measured in megahertz (1 MHz = one million cycles/second). Useful personal computing can be accomplished with processor speeds ranging from 120 MHz to more than 200 MHz; for casual personal use, 133 MHz is a minimum to prevent edginess. BOFIB.

When computers are connected to other computers, a type of information system architecture is created called "client-server" architecture.

Size

Computers used to be classified rather arbitrarily, with terms such as "supercomputer," "minicomputer," and "microcomputer." These terms are now passé, and you should adopt trendier terminology to appear erudite. Large computers are often called "mainframes." Mainframes are usually connected to devices called "terminals" or, more derogatorily, "dumb terminals," which users manipulate to enter and retrieve data.

Terminals

They are called "dumb" because they consist of only a monitor and a keyboard and are without a CPU. The terminal therefore does no computations itself, but it does enable the user to manipulate programs on the mainframe host. If a true computer, with a CPU, is linked to a mainframe, it can be induced to act in a brainless fashion so that it can function just like a dumb terminal. This is called terminal emulation.

Client/Server

When computers are connected to other computers, a type of information system architecture is created called "client-server" architecture. The computer that sends information to another computer is called the server. The receiving unit is called the client. Both computers have CPUs and can perform computations, and usually they can both act as either client or server. (The linking of computers is covered in greater depth in Chapter 4.)

Personal Computer

Several clarifications about computers are in order, because one does not want to be caught off guard. A personal computer is one specifically designed for individual use. The owner determines the programs that will be run and sets preferences for use. The initialism PC refers specifically to the original IBM product designed for this purpose, in distinction to Apple Macintosh systems, which function in a similar fashion but run on a different platform.

There are numerous other pieces of hardware within the boxes commonly referred to as computers, but they are not directly involved in actual computing and so receive the title of peripheral device.

Platform

The term "platform" refers to a combination of specific hardware and the special operating software that runs it; Apple hardware requires Macintosh operating software to run it, and this platform is not able to use software (such as Windows and OS-2) developed for PCs. Likewise, Macintosh programs cannot yet be run on PCs. This is the essence of the term *compatible software*, meaning that programs are compatible with—i.e., can be run on—selected devices.

Other Personal Computers

Laptop computers and notebook-sized computers are small portable units. They have multimedia capability, CD-ROM drives, SVGA displays, internal modems, and a host of features that are transforming executive airline travel. (It is all right to send them through the airport x-ray security screen.) *Personal Digital Assistants (PDAs)* are even smaller computers with more limited capabilities, generally used for personal schedule management. Some can produce a mean spreadsheet and load a vicious game of "Tetris". *Workstations* are beefed up or "super" PCs intended for individual use but with a specific work purpose. They usually have bigger or faster components than home PCs.

Another term to know is *clone*. If an original manufacturer of a platform (hardware plus operating system) reveals the technical specifications for the design, structure, and operation of its system (such generosity is called *open architecture*), other businesses can copy, improve, or modify the design and create a "clone" that can run any programs that can run on the original system. Because IBM developed its PC with open architecture and Apple did not, the consumer computer world has long been divided into PCs (IBM plus clones) and Apples. (This has changed only very recently, and Apple clones are now emerging.) Any discussion about which platform is preferable, like discussion of religion and politics, is to be avoided at all costs.

Peripherals

There are numerous other pieces of hardware within the boxes commonly referred to as computers, but they are not directly involved in actual
computing and so receive the title of *peripheral device*. Some peripheral
devices may actually be composed of chips and micro-electronics, such as
sound cards and *video cards*, but, even though they process bytes, they are
not the motherboard and hence are considered "peripherals."

The only items lower on the hardware food chain are network components that simply transmit data without transforming or manipulating it.
(Some words of caution: Don't offend the telecommunications department by explaining its position on the food chain. It can drop you harder than a Lawrencium bowling ball on Jupiter.) The classic peripheral
device is a printer, which converts electronic data into images on paper;
they come in numerous varieties (dot matrix, laser, ink-jet, and thermal
transfer), and printer drivers in your computer tell the specific printer
how to layout and display information on the page. Simply printing
exactly what you see on your computer screen is called *WYSIWYG*, meaning what you see is what you get.

Mice, Monitors, Modems, Scanners

Other examples of peripherals are disk drives, which manipulate data for
storage but not computation; input devices such as the keyboard and
mouse that submit information to the computer; *monitors* (the television-
like screens on which the computer displays images); *modems,* which are
responsible for preparing digital information from the computer for
transmission over phone lines; and *scanners*, which image text or graphics and convert them into digital formats that can be seen and manipulated on the monitor.

At this point, you may be beginning to feel the stirrings of vocabulary
superiority and "info-arrogance." Even now, with a grasp of bits, bytes,
CPUs, motherboards, and megahertz, you could comport yourself well at
the Microsoft reception. And you always have the BOFIB fallback if you
don't quite get some arcane term. But there are a few more concepts related to computer hardware to be mastered before tackling software. These
additional items will provide polish to the information system persona.

Hardware Data Storage

Computers need to "store" bits of data for use by the motherboard,
because the purpose of the CPU is to compute quickly. The storage of bits
of data is accomplished by allowing electrical signals to make impressions
on an electromagnetic substance, such as magnesium oxide, in much the
same fashion that they alter bit switches on a silicon chip. The substance

is coated on plastic in the form of tape, such as on a cassette tape or a *disk*. The hardware that writes and reads the signals to and from the storage medium consists of a "drive," which moves the medium, and a "head," which does the writing and reading. These drives are usually given letter designations—A:, C:, D:. Each drive is analogous to a file cabinet.

Disks

There are several types of disks: hard disks, floppy disks, compact discs, and what are now called digital versatile discs.

The hard disk is usually resident in the computer housing at the location labeled the C: drive. This is the main data storage medium for computers, and it commonly consists of several plastic magnesium oxide-coated platters stacked together. The hard disk can hold relatively large amounts of data, anywhere from 500 megabytes to 5 gigabytes. BOFIB. Information is written to the hard disk by a process called "saving." You save as you work. This results in logically related information (daily schedule updates, for example) being saved noncontiguously. This separation of data results in something called *fragmentation*, which in advanced stages can make the computer perform less swiftly than desired. The only reason to mention this here is to afford you the opportunity to ask your technical computer support people to "defragment" your hard disk, which will permanently impress them with your astounding breadth of knowledge. (They may, of course, wonder why you didn't realize that the command is available from your own keyboard on your new state-of-the-art system.)

The hard disk is usually resident in the computer housing at the location labeled the C: drive. This is the main data storage medium for computers, and it commonly consists of several plastic magnesium oxide-coated platters stacked together.

Floppy disks are pliable plastic platters coated like the hard disk but used singly and inserted into the A: drive of most computers. They come in two sizes (3.5 and 5.25 inch diameter) and hold only up to 2.8 megabytes of data per disk. By the way, the 3.5 inch floppy disks aren't very floppy at all. In fact they are pretty hard, but don't embarrass yourself by calling the *help-desk* to discuss problems with your "hard disk" if this is what you are referring to. People talk. Floppy disks start out in an "unreadable" state. In order for the drive head to record data on them, *formatting*, the process of making grooves and sectors (like record tracks and pie-slices) that act like maps onto which the data will be etched, must occur.

The other kind of data storage medium of importance is the optical disc, also referred to as the compact disc (CD). These are different from other disks

Hardware — Break it will a hammer

Computers = innards
& peripheral devices

Accept data input

CPU — central processing unit
Silicon micro processor
& micro-electronic
pathways

↓

electrical energy

↓

makes ⊕ + ⊖ impulses
& value changes in
switch.

Tiny switch in ⊕ or ⊖ state
(on or off)

~~energy~~ energy can
mean 0 (off) & 1 (on)

Binary digit (BIT).
Package 7 Bits is a byte.
32 - bit or 64 - bit
(30 FiB

because they are spelled with a "c" (for no good reason that I am aware of) and because they are coated with a thin layer of aluminum and lacquer on the side that has data etched into the plastic in the form of microscopic pits. A laser head shines a very sharp beam of light on the disc and senses the reflected energy from its surface, which varies according to the sequence and the number of pits. The photo-detector and microelectronics in the head convert the variably reflected light into bits of digital data.

The most familiar of these discs is the CD-ROM (*compact disc-read only memory*), which can be read by the computer but not written to. These hold truly wonderful amounts of data (up to 6 gigabytes) and, when used with video and sound cards, confer "multi-media" capability to the computer system. (Multi-media means one can view movies, listen to music, and play computer games; essential for executives.).

Digital Versatile Disc

To be viewed as being extremely in vogue, bring up this next generation of optical disc technology at your earliest opportunity. The digital versatile disc (DVD) can store up to 14 times more information than current CDs and can play it back at a rate of 11 million bits per second. This rate is equivalent to a 9X CD-ROM capability; current CD-ROM drives on home PCs run in the range of 2X to 12X.

DVDs are pitted on two surfaces, and the pits are half the size of those on current CDs, yielding a data spiral 11 kilometers long. Associated new formatting methods further facilitate recording of more information per pit. With technology that actually allows layering of the pit surface, storage of upward of 17 gigabytes of data per disc is quite feasible. This means one DVD not only can hold an entire movie, but also could store different languages of dialogue, different cuts and camera angles, and ultimately Dolby-type theater quality sound encoding.[1]

Sub-Micron Miniaturization

Even beyond the storage capacity of DVD is holographic data storage technology. And as you read this, techniques are emerging that allow bit encoding by the distribution of individual atoms (helium) at extremely low temperatures. Inducing placement and predictable changes in atomic particles will dominate technology in the future.

Memory

Between hard disk storage and the motherboard is another important microprocessor card. The random access memory (RAM) card functions as a critical reservoir of data. It's what keeps computer programs and information instantaneously accessible for the CPU and you.

If the CPU had to read stored data on the hard disk directly, piece by piece, computer operation would be so slow as to preclude use. The RAM card pulls data into a kind of purgatory between storage and computation, making it available instant to instant for your reading pleasure and for modification. The data resident in RAM is ephemeral. If the computer loses power for any reason, the work on the RAM card goes inexorably and irretrievably to heaven (somewhat complicating the conventional notion of being "saved").

And as you read this, techniques are emerging that allow bit encoding by the distribution of individual atoms (helium) at extremely low temperatures.

RAM is measured in megabytes. Sixteen megabytes is now the minimum you need, especially if you want to be able to "multi-task." (*Multi-tasking* means you can have several software programs running on the computer at the same time.)

Many computers have special sockets called *PCM-CIA (Personal Computer Memory Card International Association)* slots into which credit card-sized boards can be inserted to increase RAM capacity to as much as 200 megabytes. BOFIB. The amount of RAM one has on one's system is second only to the size of the hard drive in impressing others with one's hardware, but only slightly ahead of the braggadocio surrounding the speed of one's CPU.

Anything Else?

Information system hardware components don't do anything by themselves, except break. They require instructions telling the computers and peripheral devices what to do. We go there next.

Nothing you can't spell will ever work.—Will Rogers, American humorist, 1924.

Reference

1.   Bell, A. "Next-Generation Compact Discs." *Scientific American* 275(1):42-6, July 1996.

Chapter 3

Computer Software

"Software code, like laws and sausages, should never be examined in production."—
Edward Tenner, American author, 1996.

A hammer can break hardware but not *software*. This is because software is intangible. It is made up of electronic signals configured to direct computer microprocessors and electronics in a defined fashion. The nature and sequence of these desirable "instructions" for the hardware are determined by human "programmers," also called *developers*, who use special *programming language* to prepare the directions. They conceive a plan in their brains for a set of desired computer actions and then translate them into the bytes of code necessary for the computer to understand.

Software Languages

Developers begin their excellent adventure by structuring thoughts and recording them in what is called "high-level" programming language, which looks a little like natural human writing (you could recognize many words among the symbols). This language outlines *algorithms*, which are rules that define a path that guides a process to a logical end point.

There are two families of high-level coding language: the "procedural" family and the "object-oriented" family. I know this information makes some readers want to skip to the next chapter, hit the links, or get some latte, but someone important is going to ask you if you are object-oriented, and they will not be referring to your impressive personal belongings.

High-Level Coding Languages

The "procedural" family of coding language is based on an information framework (imagine an entire skeleton) and a set of procedures (picture muscle groups). The framework is manipulated by the procedures to produce purposeful motion. Examples of procedural languages (for your IBM continental breakfast) include Pascal, C, FORTRAN, COBOL, and BASIC.

The "object-oriented" family of programming language uses commands that act like little functional units (think about an entire elbow or knee joint, with all its relevant muscles, tendons, and cartilage) that can be assembled to elicit complete computer actions. Objects are models of "things," consisting of bundles of data packaged with behavior.

The "object-oriented" family of programming language uses commands that act like little functional units (think about an entire elbow or knee joint, with all its relevant muscles, tendons, and cartilage) that can be assembled to elicit complete computer actions.

These objects can interface with one another in what are called *object data models (ODMS)* and can have parent and child relationships with objects that contain more (parent) or fewer (child) data or behavior attributes. The objects themselves can come in varieties (data object, user interface object, and process object, as examples) and can themselves be bundled into groups of objects plus interfaces called "armor-plated objects." These armor-plated objects can, in turn, interface with one another in what are called *components*.

There are presently two major technologies called, OLE and CORBA, that handle these "components." You may wish to knowingly nod your head when you hear the terms *component object model (COM)* (which is the technical underpinning of OLE) and *distributed component object model (DCOM)*, which facilitates use of objects over networks. If you wish to really be trendy, you can bring up *Active X*, which carries object programs and interactive data fields to computers accessing servers over the Internet (see Chapter 4).

There are many benefits to object-oriented programming, not the least of which is the ability to combine, mix, match, and reuse portions of the code, much like interlocking puzzle pieces. Examples of object-oriented languages are C++, SmallTalk, Java, and FORTH.

Either of the two families is capable of creating a miserable product. The procedural family misfits may have bad bones, lumbago, malfunctioning muscles, one leg shorter than the other, or anything else that can distort motion. The object-oriented creations can have a hip joint where their jaw should be, which even when working perfectly can bite itself in the rear.

Low-Level Code

Regardless of which high-level language forms Quasimodo, it must be translated into "low level" or "machine" code, in streams of bits and bytes, for the computer to read and act on. This translation from high-level to low-level language is accomplished by software called a compiler, whose duty is to build the human language into atomic bits comprehensible to the CPU.

The high-level language is sometimes called the *source code*. Source code is important because you really want to own it, especially if you are in a co-development effort with a software vendor. If you do not own the source code, you cannot maintain or enhance the application it invokes. Consumers do not generally own the source code. (Having braved this discussion, you will be relieved to know that you need to bandy about only two terms: "object-oriented" and "C++." Act as if everything else is beneath you. Ok, use "java" too.)

Software Programs

The bytes of software that are "compiled" constitute a "module." Modules exist in a caste system of sorts, with the primitive "stub" module at the bottom. Above the stub are layers of other more sophisticated, but still incomplete, modules, up to the esteemed transaction, or T-level module, which can actually process a transaction. When modules reach a certain useful threshold size, a program is born. Some programs do things to and for the computer that are really "under the covers" as far as the user is concerned. This kind of program is called operating system software. The other kinds of programs are visibly useful to humans. They are called *applications*.

Examples of applications would be WordPerfect™ for text management, Excel™ or Lotus™ for spreadsheets, or DOOM 2™ for mayhem. The form of an application that is "run" by the computer is called the *executable*. A little subset of an application that can do a set of things in and of itself is called an "applet."

Files

Software programs and other computer information are stored in convenient places for use by you and/or the computer. These places are called *files*, and there are two major types: those that contain programs and those that contain data.

One can personally name data files with recognizable titles so that you can find them in current operating systems, but, despite the intuitive names you give them, they will still be identified by the computer via an automatically assigned extension abbreviation. An executable program file, for example, has the extension ".exe" (Microsoft Excel.exe). A text file created on a word processing program may be called "confusing.txt," meaning text, or "confusing.wpd," meaning a WordPerfect™ document. Graphic image files, like photographs or drawings, can be "something.bmp," or "something.jpg," or "something.gif," and on and on. Particularly large files are sometimes called "directories," which are like hanging file folders into which you stuff multiple smaller files. A file is like a manila folder, a directory is the file drawer, and the disk drive is the file cabinet.

The data in the files are stored in the form of databases, which come in several forms. Flat file databases allow users to work with only one data table at a time, whereas relational databases such as Sybase™ and Oracle™ allow multiple tables to be worked with simultaneously. A new type of database called "object-oriented " manages concepts with multiple attributes and relationships to other concepts often referred to as a knowledge base. (If you really want to flex your muscles, ask someone in your information systems department if the database being used is relational or truly object-oriented. Then call for a wet clean up.)

The operating system software prepares the computer to receive your commands. It manages files, drives peripheral devices, directs memory allocation, and guides interactions with applications.

ASCII

There are some standard formats for representing and communicating written information via computer, the common one you need awareness of being ASCII, which is the initialism for "American National Standard Code for Information Interchange."

Operating System Software

Let us return for one more agonizing moment to operating system software. This is the programming that controls basic computer functions that are critical to everything working correctly. The operating system software prepares the computer to receive your commands. It manages *files*, drives *peripheral devices*, directs memory allocation, and guides interactions with applications. There are several examples of operating systems that you must be able to talk about to be chic. Windows and Macintosh are commonly recognized, but you should add *DOS*, and *OS-2 Warp* (soon to be Merlin) to your lexicon, and *UNIX* if you are really in the know. I will leave it up to you to look these up in the glossary. If we speak at a future conference, it would be a great source of pride for both of us if you could tell me what UNIX stands for.

Software Use

When the computer is initially powered up, it self-initiates its operating system software, monitors its resources and peripherals, and steels itself for applications in a process called a *boot*. When this occurs as the system is turned on, it is called a "cold boot" (or a "hard boot"); when the process is restarted while the computer is already running it is a "warm boot" (or a "soft boot"). Either way, a seemingly interminable wait is necessary before you can do anything, unless you have religiously followed the principles of *BOFIB*.

Crashes

Warm boots are initiated by depressing the Ctrl-Alt-Del keys on the keyboard simultaneously. This is necessary when a program you are running gets stuck or fails and cannot recover. This bad thing is called an ABEND (abnormal end of task). It is the horrifying moment when you realize that any work you have done that is not saved to the disk is lost, forever. Referred to as a *crash*, a "bomb," a "hose," or a "lock-up," the ABEND is bad, but it's not the worst thing that can happen.

Another kind of "crash" is called a hard disk crash, where the head of the disk drive impales itself on the delicate disk surface, permanently obliterating the byte impressions stored there and causing irretrievable information loss.

Core Dump

As long as the foibles of software are being revealed, it is advisable to get most of them out of our system so we can end on a positive note. A *core dump* occurs when software evacuates a large amount of data, never to be seen again. A *defect* in code refers to failure of the software to perform as expected, which will be more fully addressed later in association with computer project development. A *bug* is an idiosyncrasy in a program that fouls things up, sometimes because of a mistake in high-level language but sometimes because of a spontaneous mutation of the low-level code that occurs on a bit level. Fixing (exterminating) bugs is called *"debugging."*

Viruses

Viruses are software program fragments designed to damage computer data or processes. They are communicable, traveling on floppy disks or over phone wires from host to host. They can infect a system and remain hidden, or latent, until a "time-bomb" program within them detonates.

One particular kind of virus, originally called a *worm* (having nothing to do with an applet), originally appeared in 1988 on the Internet. Its creator claimed that it started as well-intentioned software designed to figure out the size of the *Internet* itself but that it contained a bug causing it to replicate itself endlessly, clogging and paralyzing the computers it infected. Since then, viruses of many kinds have been identified. Several are reviewed here, just for fun.

As explained above, viruses are cleverly designed code segments that attach to and utilize software running on the host computer to wreak havoc. They can camouflage themselves, carry passwords along with them, and manifest themselves at varying times with varying intensity. Some viruses alter data within a system, as did the one that shut NASA down for a brief time in 1990. Others, such as the Friday the 13th Virus discovered in 1988, become active on a certain date or time, suddenly slowing computer processing and erasing disks. Strains of this particular beast have also been noted on Columbus Day and are sometimes called "datacrime" variants.

Viruses are software program fragments designed to damage computer data or processes.

The Flambé virus, discovered in 1988 (a good year for epidemics) in a consulting firm in California, altered the electron beam scanning rate in a computer monitor to the point where a conflagration occurred.

In many cases, viruses travel in "executable"' (.exe) files, so if one downloads executable programs from a network, there is risk at the time of execution. It is advisable to download only reasonably well-known commercial *shareware* and to employ a good antivirus program on one's system. It is also wise to have *backups* of disk data in case of a viral disaster. Most virus scares are hoaxes, and most viruses are relatively innocuous even when real, but, by not downloading executable files, you can largely protect yourself from a virulent infection. (Viruses can be a source of shame, raising questions as to where one has been with the modem. Antivirus protection software is available and should be used for safe computing. It is rarely effective to blame infection on contact with a toilet seat.)

Benefits

Let us turn attention to a few of the great things software programs can do. First and foremost, they get the computer to do what the user desires, often remarkably faster and more efficiently than was possible with manual processes.

Software applications present "features," which are individual useful actions.

Software applications present "features," which are individual useful actions. If a computer screen resembles a prescription pad for ordering medications, specifying the drug name is a feature, as is designating the pharmacy to which the order should be sent. A number of features together make up a "function" (prescription writing), which in turn is part of an application (order entry).

Functions are determined by users or developers on the basis of needs and economics. Functions take into account the methods of data input, the processes to be performed, the screen displays, and the ultimate informational output from the computer.

The software of greatest importance to us as visual human beings is what determines screen displays. The most engaging of these is the *graphical user interface (GUI)*, which presents little pictures of objects (icons) and buttons and menus that can be manipulated by the keyboard and the mouse. GUI is the method used in Windows, Macintosh, and OS-2 operating systems and in the applications designed to run with them. This visual and intuitive user interaction method replaces the DOS command line, with its requirement of remembering and typing commands.

> *Functions take into account the methods of data input, the processes to be performed, the screen displays, and the ultimate informational output from the computer.*

Software also enables one to run multiple programs at the same time, known as *multi-tasking*. This means you can switch rapidly from DOOM2™ to Flight Navigator™ to the department budget spreadsheet. It also enables protection of work from prying eyes, setting of personal preferences and *defaults* (items set up just for you), and customization of the *desktop* (the opening display of icons for your use).

Software makes things happen with *real-time processing*, as one does them, rather than having to wait for results (batch processing). Some programs can even remember to "save" or *back-up work*, while others call on themselves automatically when they sense the need by a process called *recursion* or spin off actions using instructions called *daemons*.

Software can create sounds and video on sound and video cards, recognize speech, manage security, and simulate all kinds of things better discussed in the hot tub at a team-building meeting.

Speech Recognition

A rapidly developing and nearly usable technology called "speech recognition" enables computers to record human utterances and automatically translate them into written language or software navigation commands. This is different from simple voice digital recording, which stores the voice on the hard disk for playback through a sound card. In specific business domains, where similar words and phrases are used repeatedly, speech recognition has been useful for some time. It generally requires training the computer to recognize voice phonetics, but thereafter it can be operator independent. Until recently, it has required noncontinuous speaking to function properly so if you .... talk .... like .... this .... it......... works .... pretty .... well. Unfortunately, continuous speech has been more challenging, with syntax, grammar, homonyms, and mispronunciations confounding matters.[1] Very recently, continuous speech recognition programs have emerged that work quite well for specific domains (radiology is a notable example). The new technology holds promise for facilitating entry of dictated material into medical records, but in and of itself it will neither refine, standardize, nor render more intelligible communications so recorded. The image of "paving the cow-path" comes to mind.

Natural Language Processing

"Natural language processing" occurs when a computer "reads" keyboard-entered text strings, separates the words or phrases into little packets (parsing), and assigns computer codes to the individual packets, thereby codifying the text for storage, analysis, and retrieval. A recent study has shown some early utility of natural language processing in the form of identifying key utterances in certain domains (radiology, again), and in at least one case the process rivaled the capabilities of humans to decipher and identify terminology in the same text.[2] Unfortunately, this says as much about the poor quality of human communications as it does about natural language processing.

One of the computer's most critical functions is to store and manipulate data entered by users, but it can only do so if the information is coded in a form that the computer can understand. The language that humans enter by typing or dictating is not coded and is referred to as "free text." The words and concepts contained in such text have no meaning to the machine. If one has associated software codes with the words ahead of time, however, and if the user chooses these words from a drop down menu or from a list on the screen, the computer knows what to do with them and can exercise its computational power over them. The ultimate system situation, which may not be too far in the future, would be one in which a torpid user could dictate information in his or her usual verbose and sloppy manner, with *speech recognition* translating the words into text. This would be followed by the computer's performing natural language processing on the text (perhaps even real-time as the user dictates) and translating the text into coded data. This is desirable because it means that the human does not have to organize, structure, contain, or accurately synthesize thoughts in order to have them all available for analysis in a coded form.

Artificial Intelligence

Artificial intelligence (AI) is a label given when an inanimate machine makes a decision to take action independent of the cognitive intention of the human user. Also called "decision support," because it requires the element of decision to differentiate it from the millions of other automatic actions computers take, AI is clearly in everyone's future, and one of its early invocations is in the form of alerts and reminders.

The actions the machine takes are based on instructions within the software that cause the computer to search for a specific set of data, make comparisons of the data, and draw conclusions based on programming rules. The rules are called *logic modules*, and they are authored by humans, but they give the impression that the computer thought of what to do next (which it really did). These rules can be invoked in real time while one is using a program (synchronous) or after completion of a task at a later time (asynchronous).

The whole area of AI is perhaps one of the most frightening aspects of new software development for users, who see their expertise and positions in the workforce being threatened.

Anything Else?

The functional combination of software with hardware is the basis of the information revolution, and therefore the understanding gained from these two chapters alone is a strong foundation for further growth. Much of the vernacular one requires to obtain a credible facade of "techno-ciliousness" has been obtained, but understanding how these components are linked to one another and how these linkages relate to enterprise structure requires absorption of some verbiage on the subject of networks.

The sad thing about artificial intelligence is that it lacks artifice and therefore intelligence.—Jean Baudrillard, French semiologist, 1987.

References

1.   Gibbs, W. " Making Sense." *Scientific American* 276(2):37-8, Feb.1997.
2.   Hripcsak, G., and others. "Unlocking Clinicial Data from Narrative Reports: A Study of Language Processing."*Annals of Internal Medicine* 122(9):681-8, May 1, 1995.

Chapter 4

Communication Networks

Is it a fact—or have I dreamt it—that, by means of electricity, the world of matter has become a great nerve, vibrating thousands of miles in a breathless point of time?— Nathaniel Hawthorne, American author, 1851.

The incredible power of new information technology has been enormously enhanced by the linking of multiple hardware devices into "networks." The extreme importance of networks in business demands more attention than is within the purview of this chapter; once one has familiarity with the basics presented here, I suggest flexing the new knowledge by obtaining a copy of *The Digital Economy*.[1] It not only is a superb book about the many aspects of networking's impact on business and society, but also can help instill confidence and foster growth after just a few fundamentals are conquered.

The all important outer layer of verbiage is next, the net gain.

Communications Media

A network is created when one hardware device is connected to another by means of a "communication medium" of some kind. Different communications media can handle various frequencies and types of data. This capacity is referred to as *bandwidth.* Wider bandwidth means faster and better communication. *BOFIB.*

Twisted Pair

Copper wire, also called twisted pair cable, is the most common medium. It is relatively inexpensive, but it is limited in bandwidth and in the distance it can span without amplifiers or repeaters. It is used for most telephone lines, but it's easily tapped (not secure) and is subject to interference by electromagnetic fields.

Coax

Coaxial cable is another common connector, often used in mainframe-terminal architecture. It is copper as well, but with higher bandwidth and better insulation against electromagnetic interference. It is quite impressive to ask someone if their coax is *baseband* (transmits only one channel of data) or *broadband* (transmits many bands or channels, such as voice, data, and video, simultaneously). Coaxial cable is also easily tapped and is therefore risky from a security standpoint.

Fiberoptic

Bandwidth is predicted to rise up to 1,000 times more than current capacity within the next 10 years, meaning that it is very likely that the network itself will become the dominant technologic entity, with computers simply becoming network communication facilitators.

Fiberoptic cable carries energy in the form of light waves rather than electrical signals. It can cover much greater distances and has a far greater bandwidth and higher speed of transmission than copper media. It is difficult to tap, very resistant to interference, and preferable in areas in which the environment may be a hazard (moisture, corrosives, extreme voltage fluctuation, lightning risk, etc.)

Energy waves of various kinds (radio-frequency, infrared, microwave, etc.) are other media that are used to connect networks via wireless broadcast over long distances. Such broadcasts are easily intercepted and are therefore not secure, unless they have undergone *encryption*.

Bandwidth is predicted to rise up to 1,000 times more than current capacity within the next 10 years, meaning that it is very likely that the network itself will become the dominant technologic entity, with computers simply becoming network communication facilitators.

Analog versus Digital

Data can be passed over communications media in one of two signal forms: *analog* or *digital*. Analog signals are "continuous." They possess an infinite number of gradations. Sound, for example, is a continuous wave of energy with varying frequencies and with an infinite number of points along the wave. Because this is reflective of actual life situations, it is called analog (analogous to real).

Analog waves tend to lose signal intensity and to degrade over distance, which means that amplifiers must be used along communication lines to boost intensity if the receiver is to understand or interpret the signal. Most phone companies use this amplification technology to send voice and data over lines. Unfortunately, the amplification process amplifies not only signals but also noise, which increases signal degradation. This degradation is relatively innocuous for voice transmission but can be problematic for more precise data transmission.

If a continuous analog sound wave were to be broken up into 100 pieces, and the frequency within each puzzle piece sampled, the process of "digitization" would have been started. Each little puzzle piece could be converted into a specified number of *bits* or *bytes* to represent its sample characteristic, thus becoming digital data that the computer can manipulate.

When connections such as this are established within a building or a department, the system is referred to as a local area network (LAN).

A computer can take the digitized bytes and reassemble them in sequence, with the resultant signal being similar but not identical to the analog one initially sampled. The smaller, more numerous, and more compact the digital samples, the more closely the digital wave resembles the analog one. This same process can be applied to the colors or densities or degree of grayness of a visual image. The digital data can be transmitted over communications *media* just as are the analog signals, but amplification of the signals is not employed to maintain the data intensity. Rather, the bytes are periodically received, sampled, and repeated with fresh intensity and with little to no degradation, leading to cleaner and more precise data transmission.

A network may link a computer to a printer, to a series of peripheral devices, or to other computers; these devices are called "nodes." A diagram of the links and nodes describes the *network topology*. More detail on network topology will afflict you in a moment, but first absorb some generalities.

Local Area Network

When connections such as this are established within a building or a department, the system is referred to as a *local area network (LAN)*. Local area networks, which are extremely common, are generally accomplished with *hard-wiring* between devices, meaning direct node-to-node connections with wire or cable.

Buildings that have been constructed with cable wiring in the walls even before devices are planned, purchased, or deployed are called "smart" buildings. In general, LANs do not require phone lines for communication or information sharing and reside in what is considered a "local environment."

Wide Area Network

If phone lines or other media are required for communication, as opposed to wires dedicated solely to the hardware devices, the network is called a *wide area network (WAN)*. Either a LAN or a WAN can use any kind of medium for connection, so use of the terms isn't necessarily precise; rather they indicate how relatively contained the whole mess is. Some

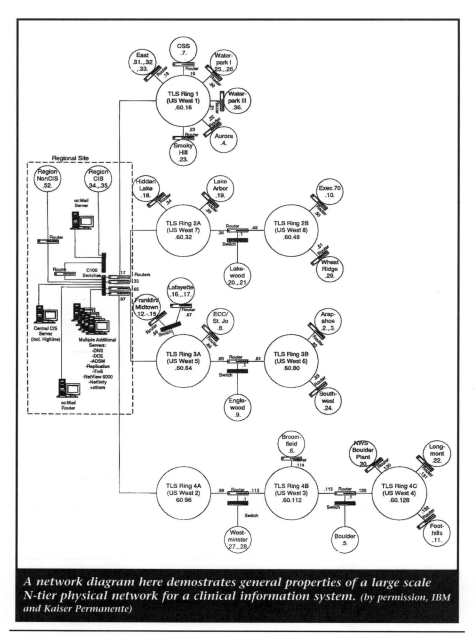

A network diagram here demostrates general properties of a large scale N-tier physical network for a clinical information system. (by permission, IBM and Kaiser Permanente)

refer to WANs only when a network spans more geography than a single metropolitan area, reserving the term metropolitan area network (MAN) for mid-sized linkages.

From a user perspective, the distinction is moot, but the technical support and telecommunications people need to be able to tell which one is down on a moment-to-moment basis. You may also hear the term *intranet*, which refers to an extensive network across many geographic locales within an enterprise. The intranet is different from the *Internet*, which is a massive connection between entities and will be discussed shortly. An *extranet* is an intranet that allows access to portions of the internal information by a verified user from "outside."

> *Client-server architecture exists where a larger computer (the server) is connected to other computers (clients), which may in turn be linked to even more computers (third-tier clients).*

Network Architecture

Configuration, structure, and connections of hardware (*computers, routers, bridges*, network connectors, *peripherals*, etc.) constitute basic *information system architecture*. In this usage, the term refers to a more complex level of network topology. Experts in system architecture, however, also use this term to describe complicated relationships and interactions of communication paths, software, and machine and human interfaces. One can hardly go wrong, therefore, asking someone about his or her information system architecture.

Mainframe architecture is most familiar, made up of a single big *central processing unit* with multiple *dumb terminals* wired into the host. The terminals that the users manipulate to enter and retrieve data in this case have no brains (CPUs) and therefore cannot be "clients" (although some have challenged this, pointing out clients who have no brains).

Client-server architecture exists where a larger computer (the server) is connected to other computers (clients), which may in turn be linked to even more computers (third-tier clients). Each client and each server must have a CPU. A rule of thumb is that a computer that sends information to another computer is a server, and one that receives information from another computer is a client. A computer can be both client and server at the same time.

Very recently, a new breed of network computer, called a *thin client*, which, like other thin things, is viewed as highly desirable in some industries, has made its appearance. Thin clients are pretty smart (they have a CPU), but they can't do much on their own because they can't remember (store) programs. They have local processing and presentation capabilities but no disks, and they therefore rely on host computers (servers) to provide applications and data needed to perform their magic. They are also called NCs (network computers). This means that regular clients are fat and smart, terminals are skinny and dumb, and thin clients are fit but forgetful (and very attractive...financially). One wants client-server architecture for most applications; fat or thin is a matter of taste and cost.

Network Components

It is useful to dissect networks into key components to simplify a complex subject. This enables one to cull the minimum number of terms needed to display command of the entire domain, which is important because most business communication, efficiency, growth potential, and frustration can be attributed to networks.

Connection Devices: Modems

Modems are *peripheral devices* that convert digital information from a computer into analog signals for transmission over standard phone lines. They also convert the analog signal back to digital for computer use. As the technology in the phone industry changes and digital repeaters rather than analog amplifiers along lines become the norm, modems will vanish.

Thin clients are pretty smart (they have a CPU), but they can't do much on their own because they can't remember (store) programs. They have local processing and presentation capabilities but no disks, and they therefore rely on host computers (servers) to provide applications and data needed to perform their magic.

A current communication technology called *ISDN (integrated services digital network)* is rapidly advancing in America. This new system transmits voice, digital, and other data with complete digital end-to-end circuits (no modem needed) and with significantly increased *bandwidth* compared to current phone lines.

Modems are assessed on the basis of the speed with which they can convert and send data, measured in *bauds*. A baud is a unit of measure that describes the number of bits of data per second that can cross a line. The modem you obtain should be rated at 28,800 baud or more. *BOFIB.*

There are several special kinds of modems. The fax-modem is just like a regular one except it can format information for reception by a facsimile machine. A "callback" modem receives a message, asks for a "password," hangs up, looks up an authenticated number, and calls back to improve security. Encryption modems scramble and unscramble information messages.

Bridges and Routers

The modem is only one type of device that connects hardware to communications media. There are others to be aware of, the most common of which are *bridges* and *routers*.

Bridges send groups of bytes from one network to another using "packet technology," which means that a generated electronic message is broken down into byte packets, with identifying segments enclosing the actual message packets to keep them in a decipherable group. Bridges on steroids are called *multipoint conferencing units (MCUs)*, which allow voice and video transmissions between networks, thereby enabling the torturous *video conference*.

Routers are programmable devices similar to bridges, but they often can present passwords and perform call-backs to secure a network. All one really needs to remember is that, short of a backhoe digging up a cable, bridges and routers will be the source of most network nightmares.

The performance of a network relies more on bandwidth than on the type of communications medium used and on protocols that configure data for transmission and define rules to coordinate the systems.

Dressed with this knowledge, one can command respect from peers, and probably from your information system department, but, to really shine, a few more conceptual armaments are needed.

Communication Rules

The performance of a network relies more on bandwidth than on the type of communications medium used and on *protocols* that configure data for transmission and define rules to coordinate the systems. Protocols determine which nodes should talk and which should listen, and when. The medium (alone) is not the message.

Most networks use "packet" technology. Protocols define and govern the format, sequence and method of sending and receiving the message packets. These protocols operate within conceptual "layers" of communication that have been specifically defined to allow systems with different hardware and network characteristics to communicate. These defined layers have been described as *Open Systems Interconnection (OSI)*.

OSI

OSI has seven layers, like the seven deadly sins. The top layer is called the application layer (**a**nger), which deals with the end user interface (what you see on the screen). The three layers beneath it, **presentation** (pride), session (sloth) and **t**ransport (gluttony), define the nature of the systems at each end of the connection. The bottom three layers, **n**etwork (covetousness), **d**ata-link (greed), and physical (lust), define network routing, message synchronization, and the actual bit transmission details of the process. Because it was developed and promulgated by the International Standards organization, it is sometimes also referred to as the ISO network layers. This is convenient for dyslexics.

OSI Layer	Facilitation	Example of Impact for Users
Application (anger)	Precise screen actions	What user wants to do
Presentation (pride)	Screen format	What user wants to see (SGML, HTML, etc.)
Session (sloth)	Conversing between computers	How user gets to communicate (HTTP)
Transport (gluttony)	Communication protocols	TCP/IP, ATM, etc. Communication protocols
Network (covetousness)	Communication protocols	TCP/IP, ATM, etc.
Data-link (greed)	Network protocols	Ethernet, token ring, ISDN, etc.
Physical (lust)	Communication media	Twisted pair, coax cable, RF, fiber, etc.

TCP/IP

An example of a very important communication protocol at the transport/network layers that is becoming a standard is *TCP/IP (Transmission Control Protocol/Internet Protocol)*. This is a set of rules for preparing and sending signals between computers, including those on the Internet.

An application layer protocol I am somewhat partial to is *ROSE (Remote Operations Service Element)*. This is a rule set that allows cooperation between two interacting applications. ROSE facilitates cooperation between clients and servers, but it does not know how to carry out the actual applications (much the same as an executive.)

Protocols and Media

Network performance depending on the combination of the communications medium and protocol employed.

T-lines

The communication convention in the United States is called the T-1 line. T-1 lines are actually twisted pair copper cable that are configured to transmit 24 voice or data conversations simultaneously at a speed of 1.5 million bits per second (baud). The European equivalent of T-lines are E-lines.

Contrary to general public awareness, the Internet is not all that "new."

Ethernet and Token Ring

Ethernet is a specific kind of network generally used within a building to connect computers and peripherals, usually consisting of coaxial cable and protocols for transmitting data in packets of bytes (64 bytes per packet) at a speed of 14,800 packets per second (that's in the range of ...carry the one...7.5 million baud). *Token ring* is another kind of LAN in the form of a closed ring with a protocol that passes a "token" to a device that allows it to dominate the entire bandwidth of whatever medium is being used for the time it needs to send its data, after which time it passes its token on. This amounts to shared domination, rather than just sharing, a technique you may want to explore in other areas of your business. Token ring is faster than Ethernet, handling up to 30,000 byte packets per second (15 million baud), but the important thing to remember is that Ethernet and Token ring do not communicate with each other very well.

FDDI

The current Schwarzenegger of network technology, however, is *FDDI (Fiber Digital Data Interface)*, which uses fiberoptic cable and allows transmission of a whopping 170,000 byte packets per second (8.7 billion baud).

Network Monitors

Network operations and performance are important for information system function, and there are additional pieces of hardware (such as the *sniffer*) and software (*network operating software, NOS*) that enable technicians to monitor and trouble-shoot linkages. Keeping this "nervous system" intact is a fundamental part of any kind of information system maintenance.

The Internet

Contrary to general public awareness, the Internet is not all that "new." It was created 25 years ago as a computer network linking vital government and academic computers together with the intent of creating a network that would allow continued computer access from multiple sites despite a nuclear attack. It mandated the TCP/IP standard, which has allowed for its growth into a global network of networks. The number of network host computers is rising exponentially, more than 13 million by 1997.

Before the advent of flashy, colorful, and relatively simple-to-create ways of posting images and information, the Internet was generally used to pass relatively ugly data and text files from place to place using *file transfer protocols (FTP)*; utility was primarily in the areas of electronic mail and bulletin boards. Advances in the esthetics and capabilities of the use interface OSI layers, and in particular in the application area, allowed an explosion of activity in the portion of the Internet called the World Wide Web, which is what most individuals cruise for work and play.

World Wide Web

The part of the Internet that has taken off since 1994, bringing networking out of the "ivory towers" and into the realm of the masses, is called the *World Wide Web (WWW).* You can access the world wide web using a modem and some browsing graphical interface software on your PC. You can contract with any of a multitude of small companies that provide entrance ramp servers to the "information highway," or you can use services such as CompuServe™ or America on Line™, which offer their own browsing software products in addition to providing connection to the Web.

Because of standards that have been adhered to in the presentation of data for communication on the Internet, the browsing program used to look things over on the Web doesn't matter much. The major navigation/browsing software programs (Netscape™, Microsoft Network™)

have slightly different capabilities, but the standards for displaying information objects for browsing is what has allowed the marvelous communication capabilities across the globe.

The rules and standards for displaying information take the form of "markup languages." *HTML (HyperText Markup Language)* is most common and allows one to launch from a word or picture in one document directly to another document or web page that has been programmatically linked to it. This capability is what stimulates endless wandering and hours of pleasure. *SGML (Standard Generalized Markup Language)* is a more robust meta-languages used for defining markup languages such as HTML, with appealing utility in displaying and interacting with medical data, giving realistic hope to the idea of the true global health record. There is little doubt that the Internet will allow such medical data transmission, including multimedia *telemedicine,* but agreement on common medical terminology will be important for this effort to succeed. The underlying communications protocol for these markup languages is called *HyperText Transport Protocol (HTTP).*

Some more complex but wonderful application programs allow transmission of images, sound, video, and animation. You will undoubtedly hear about Java, which is an object-oriented programming language related to C++ and is used to create network-sharable, platform-independent applets (aren't you glad you read chapter 3) that your computer executes or interacts with in real time. Under development is Inferno,[2] which could be really hot Java. The premier open architecture that can incorporate all types of data, including sound and video images from widely dispersed platforms, is based on technology referred to as *CORBA* (common object request broker architecture). The combination of Java and CORBA holds great promise for enabling a multitude of medical applications.[3] Active X is a related Microsoft technology that also facilitates real-time interaction with programs resident on servers.

The Internet has revolutionized entertainment, research, shopping, raunch, and communication and has raised interesting legal, ethical, ownership, and political issues in the new global information world. One can imagine the complexities presented by 13 million computers and literally billions of "home pages" and subject areas accessible to anyone who wants to post or read about them. Quality is a clear issue, and, because of sheer size, confusion is also problematic. In very recent times, new Web "searching" software has made its appearance and simplifies finding items (you have probably heard of Yahoo™, but there are many others (Lycos™, Magellan™, Excite™, Webcrawler™, etc.); these certainly don't get to the quality issues, however.

Firewall

Exploration of the benefits of a business connection with the Internet requires building a *firewall*— a set of physical and procedural measures designed to protect organization data stores from unauthorized viewing, stealing, or corruption. Whereas the Internet is accessible to anyone, an Intranet is protected from access via the Internet and is therefore available only to authorized users within your organization. The firewall allows connection to the Internet, without allowing breaches of your security by outsiders.

Compoacher is a term coined to refer to someone who steals from, defiles, or breaches the security of others' computer systems. The term is derived from the obsolete French pocher: to poke, thrust, or intrude. It should be used in place of *hacker*, which is inappropriate to use when referring to these criminals. Hacker should be reserved for identifying somewhat obsessed computer aficionados, generally with superior knowledge in the area.

Network and Information System Security

Thoughts of "network" and "security" should always occur simultaneously. (Actually, "network," "security," and "downtime" should constitute the thought unit.) Information system security refers to protection of your hardware, networks, storage media, and data from intrusion, theft, or damage.[4,5] There are three elements:

- Confidentiality of information (meaning that only properly authorized individuals can view it).

- Integrity of information (meaning that there is no accidental or intentional corruption of data).

- Availability (meaning authorized users can get to the information to perform their jobs).

Vulnerability

All information systems have points of vulnerability, most of which you could think of just based on your reading so far. They include physical risks (breakage, theft), natural risks (acts of God, coffee spills, dirt, static electricity), hardware/software risks (failure of security log-on software or improper components or firewalls), storage media risks (disk damage or loss), emanation risks (information can be intercepted from electromagnetic emanations from CPUs or communication media), communication risks (line breakage, tapping, or broadcast interception), and human risks.

People pose two threats, errors (unintentional corruption of data or information loss due to ignorance or laziness) and crimes (intentional violations for personal gain of some kind). The most dangerous security threats come from users who share passwords, leave sensitive information visible, divulge encryption keys, or load unauthorized software onto their computers that interferes with normal operations. A subject of paramount importance if you are a manager, which will be more completely addressed in a later chapter, is intentional sabotage of a system because the automation itself or the information it collects threatens the ego of the user or his or her sense of well-being in the company.

Threats and vulnerabilities can be lumped into three main areas: "computer security" refers specifically to protecting the data and information in the computer; "physical security" refers to protection of equipment from theft or damage; and "communications security," most relevant to networks and the reason I got off on this rant to begin with. Network security focuses on protecting data that are streaming over communication media.

The combination of standards of transmission and display with excellent cryptography suggest that even the most sensitive data, such as medical information, could be made securely and confidentially available on the Internet.

Log-On

The most familiar element of network security is *password* protection, which consists of *identification* and *authentication*. When *log on* to a system occurs, users are prompted for identification and requested to take a number of additional actions that allow the system to authenticate them. The password, wherein a private series of keystrokes are entered, is the most familiar.

Other methods of authentication include keys, cards, tokens, and something called *biometrics*. Biometrics are unique personal characteristics (fingerprints, handprints, retinal vascular patterns, voiceprints, iris characteristics, etc.) that the system can compare to a stored original to ensure integrity. There are many ways to use and choose passwords to enhance security; sharing of passwords or failure to comply with other security policies must carry severe consequences, particularly if confidential patient information is being handled. Once users realize that unauthorized individuals using their IDs and passwords can take actions legally attributable to them, they tend to be more careful. Equal in importance to security measures is the balance policies must strike between access to

Once users realize that unauthorized individuals using their IDs and passwords can take actions legally attributable to them, they tend to be more careful.

needed information and unauthorized prying, because denying individuals access to needed data can destroy operations as fast as breeches in security can.

If confidential information is to be transmitted over communication media that can be tapped or intercepted, the ancient art of *encryption* may be warranted. Encryption is the process of converting readable text into unintelligible "cipher text," which must be "deciphered" by a reverse process when it reaches its secure destination. Encryption is performed using an algorithm that applies a series of mathematical formulas in different combinations to the original text. The *algorithm* also usually employs an *encryption key* that is used as a password to lock or unlock (enable) the transformation process. The key itself must also be secured. Sometimes even passwords are encrypted.

If an organization has important data on disparate systems with different platforms, which is the case most all of the time, it is faced with the ugliest, nastiest, and most disconcerting problem of all: integration.

This has no doubt made you curious about that giant party line already discussed, the World Wide Web. Encryption has been successfully used in a number of ways to make individual data transmissions "secure" on the Internet. Some browser programs (such as Netscape) use software that is referred to as a Secure Sockets Layer (SSL) to encrypt information on command or automatically in a very sophisticated way (so called 1024 bit encryption) that would take unauthorized compoachers years to unscramble. This security is what makes it safe to do banking and to distribute credit card numbers with relative impunity over the public network. In fact, some encryption software is so sophisticated it even scares the government, which considers encryption in the same category as munitions and arms. Other examples of such confidentiality software include Pretty Good Privacy (PGP, no kidding) and Virtual Private Network (VPN). An emerging type of encryption for use over networks involves private secure methods of reading information only after one has specifically accepted responsibility for doing so. This is analogous to signing for a letter before opening an envelope (and is therefore referred to as "cryptolope" technology).

The combination of standards of transmission and display with excellent cryptography suggest that even the most sensitive data, such as medical information, could be made securely and confidentially available on the Internet. This would represent a step forward in quality of care for all patients, despite outbreaks of public hysteria on the topic. I believe electronic information in this form is more secure and confidential than the current paper medical record (the one that is never available at the time of an appointment).

Insecurity

Four important words about security. There really isn't any. The Pentagon has been broken into a quarter of a million times. Airline and HBO systems have been compoached. Banks, satellites, and the White House have been intruded on. All one can do is the best one can do.[6] There are numerous issues with respect to security and confidentiality of medical information, but I believe that, if reasonable care is taken, the availability of important health information for laudable purposes outweighs the potential vulnerability to abuse.[7,8] Organizations that track down compoachers and intruders, combined with legislation to punish offenders, will continue to evolve, but with increased stores of information comes increased potential for wrongdoing.

Anything Else?

One more enormously important thing must be comprehended. Regardless of the choice of media, routers, bridges, protocols, or configurations, computer systems may still not be able to talk to each other. If an organization has important data on disparate systems with different platforms, which is the case most all of the time, one is faced with the ugliest, nastiest, and most disconcerting problem of all: *integration.*

Lack of integration is what happens when cream-of-the-crop experts go to their silos and create great systems or purchase "best of breed programs." (Think for a moment about the overall utility of a diverse "best-of-breed" approach to a dog sled team.) Armed with understanding of the terms and concepts presented so far, one should have the mildly uncomfortable feeling that there may be substantial problems getting systems to come together.

Transport of the mails, transport of the human voice, transport of flickering pictures— in this century as in others our highest accomplishments still have the single aim of bringing men together.—Antoine de Saint-Exupéry, French aviator, writer, 1939.

References

1. Tapscott, D. *The Digital Economy*. New York, N.Y.: McGraw-Hill, 1996.
2. Rodgers, R. "Java and Its Future in Biomedical Computing." *Journal of the American Informatics Association* 3(5):303-7, Sept.-Oct. 1996.
3. Forslund, D., and others. "The Importance of JAVA and CORBA in Medicare." *Processing of AMIA Fall Symposium,* Oct. 1997, pp. 364-8.
4. Russell, D., and Gangemi, G. *Computer Security Basics*. Sebastopol, Calif.: O'Reilly and Associates, 1992.

5. Barry, B., and others. "How to Achieve Secure Environments for Information Systems in Medicine." In *Medinfo '95 Proceedings*, Greenes, R. and others, Editors, Geneva, Switzerland: International Medical Informatics Association, 1995.

6. Van Bemmel, J., and Musen, M. *Handbook of Medical Informatics.* Bohn, Germany: Springer-Verlag, 1997, pp.503-12.

7. Kluge, E. "Health Information, the Fair Information Principles and Ethics." *Yearbook of Medical Informatics*. Philadelphia, Pa.: J.B. Lippincott, 1995.

8. Cushman, R. "Serious Technology Assessment for Health Care Information Technology." *JAMIA* 4(4):259-65, July-Aug. 1997.

Chapter 5

DATA, INFORMATION, AND SYSTEMS

What is information? What are data? How does one convert business practices into information models? As in previous chapters, the emphasis here is on vocabulary and on establishing information system literacy.

Data versus Information

Small units of data, called *data elements*, are represented by *bits* and *bytes* in the computer. Recall that, in Chapter 2, a byte was compared to a musical note in a symphonic score. (If you are not musically inclined, substitute an alphabetic character for the note and imagine a book of your liking.)

If several "data elements" (notes or letters) are grouped together in a logical way, they take on more meaning and their resultant grouping is called a *data structure*. A data structure might be a chord, or a word, that could be pleasing to the ear or recognizable to the eye. The same data elements could be combined in a different way to make an awful sound or an unreadable word, so data *"validity"* is important in precisely determining the desired data structure. Data structures can be gathered into groupings that have even more meaning—a melody or a sentence—and further combined into movements or sonnets, operas or novels.

> *The point at which the data element becomes information is really up to the listener or reader and to the circumstance the data represents.*

The point at which the data element becomes *information* is really up to the listener or reader and to the circumstance the data represent. Sometimes, a single note or character is information—complete, meaningful, and relevant; other times it is just wasted ink. There are no hard and fast distinctions between data and information. If one wants or needs to hear middle C in order to do a task or to see the letter F to be able to perform a job, the byte package for middle C or letter F are information; they are relevant, useful, and presumably accurate. They are concise messages that are accessible, and they sound like all other middle Cs and look like all other Fs (they are comparable). This is an unusual instance in which data really are information. It is almost never true that more data equal more information. (The desire of some companies to produce more data has led to data pollution and not to enlightenment. This is why reports on your desk are often about as useful as a parachute that opens on impact.)

There are some subtleties to consider. A series of Fs on a report card is information, but a series of Fs in the middle of a sentence is data garbage. A middle C sounded repeatedly is data noise, unless it is chimed in a numeric fashion to indicate time. Information is really data that have been filtered or aggregated in a way that is meaningful to a user. The aggregated or filtered data must have certain characteristics to qualify as information. First and foremost, they have to be comprehensible and useful to the person who needs them. Relevant is the operational word. The data also have to be available when they are needed. They have to be accurate, in the sense that the same data aggregate always equals the same information (some call this validity), which does not necessarily imply that the information is accurate with respect to the outside environment.

Information has to contain all of the data to make the user confident that it is complete (no letters missing, correct number of beats per measure). It must also be concise and clear (not buried in text or noise). Finally, information needs to be "comparable" to other instances of the same data, ideally with the same precise meaning. A unique example of confusion in this regard is the medical term "fundus," which means the main part of the uterus to an obstetrician but a part of the eye to the ophthalmologist—same data structure, different information.

Relating Information to Business Functions

At some point, the data structure can be identified with a component in your business; such components are called *entities*. Entities are items (people, places, things, events, and especially processes) that an organization needs or uses to produce value. Entity-related "data structures" will be things one wants to record, measure, or manipulate. Only after business entities and their related data structures have been defined will information systems become helpful. A huge mistake organizations make is investment in information systems without having first "decomposed" practices into core entities. Consultants can help companies decompose entities in a directed fashion, as long as they do so *with* operations experts and not *for* them.

The Enterprise Model

The representative aggregation of all of these entities is an *enterprise model,* describing core business processes independent of organizational structure. The relative purity of the model is what allows selection or construction of a set of information generating tools that will move the business forward.

Until one understands the enterprise model and the components and processes entities relevant to the areas of desired computerization, one will be hampered in designing or developing useful applications. This is especially true for clinical processes.

The enterprise model comprises entities and their relationships. Each entity can be associated with a "data structure," and the description of these data structures in this context is called a *data model.* Data modeling can be collected in a *data dictionary*, which is a good thing for an enterprise to have for several reasons. First, its creation forces an understanding of the business itself, because before data can be modeled, entities and processes must be described. This exercise alone often reveals areas in which vast improvements can be made, information systems not withstanding. Second, it creates a standard that forces comparability, which is key for good information. Third, it serves as a guide to appropriate expenditures on information technology and architecture that will best meet the *goals* and *mission* of the organization, thus minimizing wasted efforts and eliminating unnecessary culture shock.

Metaphors have been preferred over examples up to this point because they are so much easier to appreciate, but, in this case, some examples of how an enterprise model could be developed and used to help define information needs might be very helpful.

Business organizations typically have certain core "functions" they perform. Within the core functional areas are subject areas that support the functions, and within the subject areas are the *entities* and relationships that constitute day-to-day activities. The functional areas (also called business areas) can be defined independently of the organizational

Entity-related "data structures" will be things one wants to record, measure, or manipulate. Only after business entities and their related data structures have been defined will information systems become helpful.

This exercise alone often reveals areas in which vast improvements can be made, information systems not withstanding.

structure and personnel. Functional areas might be customer relations, facilities management, maintenance and planning, financial accounting, budgeting, compensation, etc. Information management itself would be a functional area. Subject areas within each business function focus on categories aimed more at drilling down to entities and data structures. For example, within the function "business planning/administration" might be subject areas of policies/procedures, regulations, legal actions, and strategic services.

Information in a knowledge base is represented as individual concepts related to one another in a logical manner, through hierarchies of parents and children but also through meaningful links to one another (also called "semantic links").

After functions and subject areas have been defined and information needs of each subject area have been evaluated, data dependencies between areas can be established. Interdependency is common between subject areas, so you can see how quickly all of this can get out of hand. Once the dependencies are listed within subject and functional areas, they are categorized by whether they involve creation of data, reading of data, updating of data, or deletion of data. A complex matrix of all functions and subject areas is created and filled in with the C,R,U,D, designations, resulting in an appropriately named *CRUD diagram. Voilà*, you have an integrated, business-oriented view of your enterprise. The CRUD diagram, however, can only be understood by those with advanced degrees in neuroscience or astronomy. A complete, detailed enterprise model from end to end in all areas of endeavor is not suggested, because only certain parts of the analysis are needed for system planning. Even if one could model all business areas, the initial mappings would have changed by the end of the evaluation process.

In summary, global planning for useful information technology progresses from business function identification to the next lower level of subject area definition for each business area. Within each subject area, entities of importance to an endeavor are defined. These entities are then related to data objects (also called data models), which are really just the defined attributes of a data structure.[1] The data objects, their relationships, and their attributes should be denoted with standard accepted naming conventions and code sets and be documented in a "data dictionary."

System Basics

The data collected, based on the enterprise model, will be stored in *databases.* They were described in Chapter 3, but to review, simple databases, called flat files, allow work on one data table or set of data fields at a time.

Larger databases employ "relational tables" (e.g., Sybase, Oracle) that enable multiple tables or sets of fields to be worked on at one time. An emerging type of database, called "object-oriented," manages concepts with multiple attributes and relationships to other objects, which represents significant evolution from the tables construct.

A stunning way to represent data in the object-oriented structure is in something called a *blob*, which gathers a miraculous number of very important data attributes into one convenient place. This feature is one that analysts have been dreaming of for years, because it coalesces logically related elements into a form that is perfect for scientific or business enterprises.

Another remarkable method of representing data that transcends the common relational table databases so abundant in today's systems is the *knowledge base*. Information in a knowledge base is represented as individual concepts related to one another in a logical manner, through hierarchies of parents and children but also through meaningful links to one another (also called "semantic links"). A vastly superior way of representing large bodies of knowledge, such as medical terminology, this method dwarfs the capabilities of current data storage processes, because it has the ability to automatically classify data concepts on the basis of what the system knows about the concept. A knowledge base almost thinks, and in this respect is similar to a *project executive*.

Software that accesses the knowledge base data for display in the application graphical user interface allows individuals in the business who manage the knowledge base to simultaneously manage the applications without having to contact a programmer to change elements that have been "hard-coded" into the software.

Another concept of importance with respect to business databases is the central data repository (CDR), referring to the collection from peripheral servers or disparate systems of all relevant data into a single logical or physical container. Also called a "data-warehouse," it is a fundamental element of "integration."

Another concept of importance with respect to business databases is the *central data repository* (CDR), referring to the collection from peripheral servers or disparate systems of all relevant data into a single logical or physical container. Also called a "data warehouse," it is a fundamental element of "integration." More will be said about integration later, but think about the fact that integration of systems means linking computers together through *interfaces*, which can be an enormous challenge, particularly when the units are on different *platforms*.

Availability

Availability is a key element of information that generally depends on the amount of time a system, program, or network is accessible for use. Often availability is described in days by hours (7 by 24) of "up time." Other important terms associated with availability are *performance*, *reliability*, *fault tolerance*, and *maintenance*. Performance describes how quickly a system will execute its intended functions. Reliability indicates the ability of a system to perform its functions without errors, crashes, or performance problems. It is measured and reported by mean time between failures.

In rather cold terms, an information system is a series of human and automated activities whose purpose is to collect, analyze, manipulate, and communicate facts about entities in a business endeavor.

Fault tolerance refers to information system architecture that ensures maximum performance and minimal failure or downtime. Fault-tolerant systems generally require redundant storage media, power supplies, and other critical components. One type of fault-tolerant architecture is *replicated technology*, a new method of multiplying the shortcomings of mainframe computing into a network of occasionally communicating, smaller, separate computers, each of which is intended to serve as a back up for the other in the event of a *point failure*. This technology gives the impression that performance will be optimized and that takeover functions will be a distinct advantage to users, ignoring the fact that there may thousands of nonbacked-up points of failure that have nothing to do with the computers (routers, bridges, cables, protocols, etc.).

Maintenance addresses ongoing activities to support system use and to repair breakage after deployment. This means fixing bugs when they arise, updating code with enhancements, training and supporting new users, repairing equipment, monitoring networks, and tracking performance.

Redundancy, *archiving*, and *disaster recovery* also affect information availability. Redundancy is a unique term, with a meaning antonymous to the one generally acknowledged in English language dictionaries. Whereas in everyday usage redundancy means superfluous and unnecessary, in the world of data it means essential and indispensable. Because there is virtually a 100 percent chance that any data element or program can be damaged or lost (called a *disaster*), information system architects apply preventive measures by duplicating each element or program and storing it for use in the event of a problem.

Archiving is the act of moving immediately accessible data from a computer to a storage medium, such as magnetic tape or optical disc, because it has filled up the on-line capacity of the system. The archived data are still obtainable, just not in a convenient or timely fashion. Archiving is a very important practice not only to keep on-line performance optimized, but to guard against disaster. Disasters can be major, such as (acts of God) (hurricanes, earthquakes, or spontaneous combustion, also called "force majeur"), or less major, such as acts of humans) (coke spills, static electricity, or gum). Sometimes data can be recovered through a process called disaster recovery.

Information Systems

Now, back to *information systems*. They consist of users, users, users, hardware, users, software, users, networks, and users. The minor components of software and networked hardware, along with an understanding of what constitutes information, can be enormously powerful in helping reach goals. In rather cold terms, an information system is a series of human and automated activities whose purpose is to collect, analyze, manipulate, and communicate facts about entities in a business endeavor. These systems are only as strong as their weakest links, and none of these activities can be successful in the absence of trust and acceptance by humans. More simply defined, a system is a network of many variables in causal relationship with one another— within a system a variable may even have a causal relationship with itself.[2] This is especially true when the variable is a human being.

Computers may be great at crunching numbers, organizing work, and storing data. Networks are excellent at enhancing communication (when they are working). Neither of them can determine what should be collected or analyzed, or how business should change on the basis of information gathered. Computers do not equal good information, nor are they solely responsible for poor information. Information systems can help greatly with some business needs, but they will not cure human frailties, nor will the information they provide alone transform a company.

Users

To ensure success of an information system, one must do all the right technical things: requirements gathering, data modeling, architecture design, availability planning, and performance prediction. Even so, the major component of the system is still the human who interacts with it in an attempt to enter or retrieve data (or play games). The most common reason for software and system malfunctions is *user error*.

Because of the issues of availability and user error, one needs a strong division of *user services* within the information systems department. More depth on this is presented in chapter 10, but for now the understanding that user services personnel are responsible for setting up, maintaining, and troubleshooting computers and their applications for users is sufficient. The usual initial contact with user services is through the *help desk*, which functions like well-done medical triage, enabling patients to get better on their own. (This process is also called "empowerment.") The help desk is structured to allow a very frustrated and angry user, in the midst of a tumultuous schedule, to call a convenient phone number that is reliably busy. In the event that human contact is initiated, Mad's law is invoked: The degree of help delivered is inversely proportional to the caller's agitation and always approximates the value of the help attained by a busy signal.

Anything Else?

Health care managers should bear in mind that leading users, implementing technological change, dealing with information politics and resistance, and using information to maximum benefit are as important as basic understanding of the components of tools and projects in the information age. Any preconception that the concise road-map of language in this first part of the book will adequately prepare one to advance, absent an understanding of the more abstract fundamentals in Part III, should be immediately expunged. Mixing chemicals without an understanding of principles and reactions often leads to undesirable results, such as explosions.

The Sufi teaching story that introduced this book should make it clear that no disrespect is intended when I suggest that you are ready to begin the journey to the "Land of the Fools." At this point, prepared with an understanding of the watermelon, it is crucial to recognize that successful use of the new fruit to benefit your patients and business will depend on your ability to understand others and integrate difficult cultures.

Adding the bugs and glitches of software to the limits and quirks of hardware is a recipe for problems that can easily wipe out the productivity gains of any system. This need not happen, of course, but the triumphs of computing are understandibly reported more frequently then disasters that most managers would rather keep from competitors.— Edward Tenner, American author, 1996.

References

1. Bachman/ Analyze Enterprise Model Guide, Release 4.10. Bachman Information Systems, Inc., 1992.
2. Dörner, D. *The Logic of Failure*. Addison-Wesley Publishing, 1996, p. 73.

INFORMATION SYSTEMS AND ORGANIZATIONS

Part 3

The health industry is in dire need of tools and techniques for merging cultures, enhancing teamwork, and understanding differences in the new world of corporate medicine. Managing the fears that arise in times of rapid change, particularly as they relate to information technology, is essential if enterprises, including medical ones, are to evolve.

Now change seems invisible, hidden in transparent pulses in the air. The appeal of a retreat into the past is not surprising. But it's too late to go back. The new road will stretch out ahead of us regardless of our ambivalence.—Jennifer James, cultural anthropologist, 1996.

The chapters that follow are particularly important for leaders who want to facilitate cooperation among groups with disparate values, to extend their understanding of corporate structure, and to approach change management with new insight. Because intense, information-based coordination is a prerequisite for living systems, comparisons of the splendid integration and efficiency of animate organisms to the less than splendid operations of most enterprises provides some interesting possibilities for the strategic use of information systems in business.

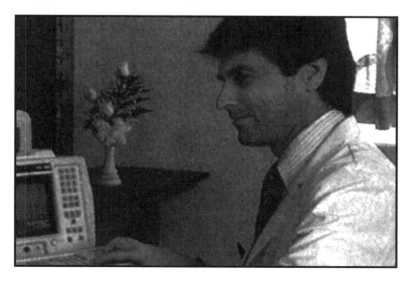

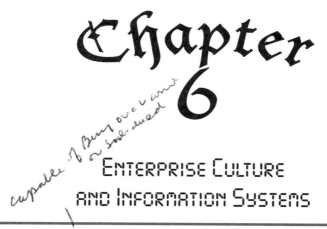

Chapter 6

ᴇɴᴛᴇʀᴘʀɪꜱᴇ ᴄᴜʟᴛᴜʀᴇ ᴀɴᴅ ɪɴꜰᴏʀᴍᴀᴛɪᴏɴ ꜱʏꜱᴛᴇᴍꜱ

Most ignorance is <u>vincible</u> ignorance: we don't know because we don't want to know.— Aldous Huxley, British author, 1950.

The use of new technology to collect and disseminate information throughout an organization can have very significant social ramifications. Just as when two countries are suddenly merged, borders between co-existing business subcultures can vanish, "currencies" can mix, and "language" differences can introduce confusion. Ideologies can clash, as can practice methods, and fears of domination and control may arise. (The term "subculture" is used here as a label for a collection of human behaviors within departments, divisions, or functional areas that are linked to one another by common tools, language, and abstract thought.) The extent to which subculture mixing hinders enterprise function and growth depends on the amount of diversity at the time of intermingling, the willingness of occupational communities to trust or compromise, and the ability of leaders to instill a common sense of purpose and a desire to cooperate in previously isolated groups.[1,2]

This brief chapter is intended primarily for managers in health care who face the challenges of getting large groups of constituents to see things the way they do and to help in building a sense of trust and common purpose. Because the case presentation in Part I of this book dealt primarily with medical opportunities in this regard, this portion uses the subcultures of informatics and management as illustrative examples.

Understanding Differences

Excellent cooperation between management and technology subcultures is essential for the development and maintenance of enterprise information systems and for the transition to a "learning organization." The importance of learning, and particularly "organizational learning," as a critical competitive advantage in today's business world, as well as alternative definitions of the term "learning organization," are elegantly addressed elsewhere.[3]

Reciprocal immersion in the vocabulary and the belief systems by both subcultures is an important step in bringing management and information system communities together, and success in harmonizing these two communities makes it much more likely that the fruits of their combined labor will be well received by numerous "tribes" of users. The following scenario illustrates some of the baseline cultural differences and emphasizes the challenges in developing new productive relationships.

The management team strongly desires a remote, primitive, off-site, outward-bound, fall-and-let-others-catch-you, conceptual, block-busting session. They want to decide on strategy and "get arms" around the issues. They want to dialogue, outline general directions, get a *mission* statement together, and bask in the wisdom of years of stable experience. They intend an informal session to exercise intuition and build trust.

The informatics community cannot understand why this process can't be done by *video conference* and is not enamored with the notion of falling. No one has ever caught them before, and they can't see why anyone would want to catch them anyway. They want a *Gantt* chart representation of the meeting plan, fingers on a keyboard, a set of well-defined problems for solution, and an *algorithm* for rules of behavior at the retreat; they have no idea what a mission statement is, but they do have a 600 gigabyte optical disc full of business data that they know would be much more effective than wisdom and body language at solving critical enterprise problems. Nothing in their world is stable, they don't believe in intuition, and they have no tangible reason to trust. (Perhaps a better start than the retreat would be to pleasantly explain that, because you read this book, they should too. Then you can all get together to point out the mistakes I made in your relative areas of expertise and everyone will begin to feel congruent happiness.)

Executives may already know that more data do not always mean more *information*, that the business cannot possibly afford constant acquisition of emerging technology, and that the same piece of information can have radically different social impacts on the organization. This knowledge, however, will be at odds with the well-intentioned beliefs of informaticists that more data always add more value, that *BOFIB* ensures company success, that every single activity in the entire business must be decomposed and diagrammed, and that information only benefits human behavior and work performance (an outlook characterized as *technocratic utopianism*[4]).

Imagine that the managers wish to embark on an automobile trip. They have excellent vision (eyesight) and knowledge about the destination, map, and road. They have no arms or legs, however, and cannot steer, accelerate, or brake. Their information technology partners are sound of body, strong, skilled, and coordinated, with cat-like reflexes, but completely blind. Taking the trip as an isolated subculture rightfully scares everyone, and mutely inhabiting the same vehicle doesn't assuage the concerns either party has about getting somewhere alive. (If one wished to extend the metaphor to health care, one might imagine that the vehicle is an ambulance with a dying patient in the back.)

> *Throughout organizations, however, there are multitudes of individuals and groups who will respond to technological change and the new flow of information in ways that are most unhealthy for the business.*

The key element of success in this situation is communication, about destination, direction, and changing conditions from the managers and about mechanical responsiveness and vehicle performance from the technologists. The better the communication and the greater the cooperative exertion of relative skills, the more likely it is that fear will abate and a happy outcome will be achieved. Any miscommunication, misunderstanding, or other interference with collaboration obviously presents a very high risk to both groups once the trip has begun. (Unfortunately, there are plenty of companies in which the information systems people only feel secure when they are trying to sew management's eyes shut, and the executives are concurrently having the function and position of the pedals changed.)

There are no hard and fast rules for cooperative operation of the vehicle, or for accomplishing the melding of cultural groups, although organization change experts and management gurus have outlined some valuable core principles for approaching the latter.[5,6] I contend that compliance with their suggestions cannot even be entertained until the divergent points of view are mutually appreciated and a basic core of shared language is established.

The merger of management and information technology subcultures provides a relatively dramatic illustration of the difficulties in achieving cooperation because of the uniqueness of their communities. Throughout organizations, however, there are multitudes of individuals and groups who will respond to technological change and the new flow of information in ways that are most unhealthy for the business. I believe that there is a unifying central concern that specifically impedes progress with information systems that is quite straightforward. I call this core dread "infobia."

Understanding Infobia

The need to collect and communicate information for the overall well-being of the enterprise means that everyone has to face a very powerful and disquieting feeling in addition to the discomfort of the incompetence associated with change. They have to come to grips with the fact that they may be judged in ways that were not possible before.

Infobia refers to the combination of two powerful fears: fear of appearing incompetent using information system technology and fear of potential harmful effects that information might have on position, prestige, or job security. Humans have strong feelings about appearing incompetent, and technological change of almost any kind means that the "changee" is going to appear incompetent at some task over which they previously had mastery (or no ability whatsoever).

Most professionals endure an educational lifetime of feeling incompetent; it's called "school." When they finally achieve a sense of competency and comfort, the last thing they want to do is go back to feelings of inadequacy. They do not want to take a new class and get a grade. They do not want to foul up on something everyone on the organization chart below them can do. Nonclinical managers are no different in this regard; they will attest that they rely heavily on human interactions to assess situations and exercise thoughtful communication (which is true), but is this really why someone else has to print or transcribe their e-mail? Or is it because they might appear incompetent if they forgot their *log-on password*, or they misused grammar, or they brought down the *network* by breaching a *firewall*?

The need to collect and communicate information for the overall well-being of the enterprise means that everyone has to face a very powerful and disquieting feeling in addition to the discomfort of the incompetence associated with change. They have to come to grips with the fact that they may be judged in ways that were not possible before. In the past, many individuals have clung to the secure belief that their value "cannot be measured" (which is different than "is immeasurable"). This attestation will be a feeble refrain in the changing climate.

Understand that, from a *user* perspective, one of three things is likely to occur as a result of new information in their area:

- They will be shown to be inadequate by good information.

- They will be shown to be inadequate by flawed information.

- Their position in the company will become less important, regardless of their personal adequacy, because of conclusions management will draw from either good or flawed information.

Because Chapter 1 focused on infobia among clinicians, it might be useful for nonclinical executive, administrative, or managerial readers to prepare themselves by imagining what their reactions would be to the introduction of a new corporate software program, called "Execution," developed by a group of doctors, that automatically measures each leader's judgment, wisdom, and vision on a day-to-day basis and reports it via e-mail to everyone in the organization.

Another metaphor may be helpful to illustrate infobia-based issues. Because business climates are changing with dramatic rapidity, a pervasive feeling of destabilization is becoming the norm for many workers. The instability is treacherous. It makes employees feel as if they are constantly in danger of being dropped into river rapids. This is disconcerting even to the strongest athletes, and it frankly terrifies those who never received their "minnow" card in swimming lessons at summer camp.

From the management perspective, the swirling water is the new world, and teaching people to survive and flow in it is a significant factor in enterprise success; information looks like life jackets.

From the management perspective, the swirling water is the new world, and teaching people to survive and flow in it is a significant factor in enterprise success; information looks like life jackets. It does not follow, however, that giving everyone a life jacket is going to make them all thrilled to jump in the river, and even more damaging is the possibility that making available with new systems information that was previously a source of special security may be experienced as taking life jackets away. Managers may be confident that the new data-driven procedures and information are critical to the business as a whole, but if they leave the responsibility for high data quality, ethical information use, and sensitive technology deployment entirely to the information services department, they should not be surprised to witness distribution of life jackets filled with lead shot.

Keeping this metaphor in mind as information-driven change is instituted will help with the prediction of when lost oars or mysteriously deflated rafts might sabotage the excellent whitewater adventure and may also help to identify people who are ill-prepared nonswimmers but paradoxically proclaiming confidence in their aquatic abilities. (They ironically may be the people formerly most valuable to the organization, with demonstrable special skills and great dedication.) It can also serve as a reminder that individuals who believe they are drowning will clutch at and pull under anything that they think might keep them at the surface. Acts of sabotage, conscious or subconscious, in the electronic world effect over half of all companies surveyed in one study.[7]

The terms Luddites and Luddism subsequently became associated with individuals phobic about new technology, particularly if the new technology appears to infringe on job security.

The most formidable elements of infobia rampant in medical culture are more completely reviewed in Chapter 1. Because the magnitude of all this is a little upsetting, I offer the following historical observation as encouragement before proceeding:

In England during the early stages of the Industrial Revolution (1811-1816), the mechanized weaving loom made its appearance in factories of textile-producing communities, notably Nottingham. Companies that used the new looms could produce garments at much less expense and in far greater quantities than those that persisted in using artisans and craftsmen for the process.

Loom machines began to break down mysteriously with increasing frequency, and the equipment failures were blamed on the evil Ned Ludd, who was rumored to have broken the first mechanized loom in around 1799. King Ludd, or General Ludd, as he was known, was probably fictional, but he became the rally leader for a band of alienated ex-weavers who became increasingly violent and aggressive saboteurs, opposing the new technology and becoming known as the Luddites. In April 1812, a mill in Lancastershire was vigorously defended from a Luddite expedition by hired soldiers, after which time the mill owner's home was attacked and things went from bad to worse.

Machinery continued to be smashed and factories burned. Suspicious murders and kidnappings occurred off and on, particularly when economic times were hard. British government involvement; a number of trials, jailings, and hangings; along with more prosperous economic times, eventually diminished Luddite activities and ended the violence.

The terms Luddites and Luddism subsequently became associated with individuals phobic about new technology, particularly if the new technology appears to infringe on job security. Radical Luddites are sometimes said to hold to the doctrine of *mosoneism*, which is extreme hatred of change or of anything new.

The Luddites have a home page in the Internet.

Change happens.

Anything Else?

Dealing with infobia means first acknowledging it. In order to manage it, some thought revisions about traditional enterprise structure and change processes are very helpful.

Millions of workers have lost their jobs as a result of downsizing, right-sizing, outsourcing, and reengineering. The resurgence of insecurity in the workplace has reawakened the fear of joblessness in many workers in all fields. Fear makes companies less competitive and adaptive, and causes workers to become less, rather than more productive.— Geoffrey James, U.S. Author, 1996.

References

1. Schein, E. *Organizational Culture and Leadership*, 2nd Edition. San Francisco, Calif.: Jossey-Bass Publishers, 1992.
2. Lorenzi, N. and Riley, R. *Organizational Aspects of Health Informatics: Managing Technological Change*. New York, N.Y.: Springer-Verlag, 1995.
3. Tapscott, D. *The Digital Economy*. New York, N.Y.: McGraw-Hill, 1996.
4. Davenport, T., and others. "Information Politics." *Sloan Management Review* 34(1):53-65, Fall 1992.
5. Lorenzi, N., and others. "Antecedents of the People and Organizational Aspects of Medical Informatics: Review of the Literature." *JAMIA* 4(2):79-93, March-April 1997.
6. Kaplan, B. "Addressing Organizational Change Issues into the Evaluation of Medical Systems." *JAMIA* 4(2):94-101, March-April, 1997.
7. Ernst and Young Survey, *Toronto Financial Post*, Dec. 15, 1994, p.6.

Chapter 7

Enterprise Structure and Information Systems

Nature is a self-made machine, more perfectly automated than any automated machine. To create something in the image of nature is to create a machine, and it was by learning the inner working of nature that man became a builder of machines.—Eric Hoffer, U.S. philosopher, longshoreman, 1973.

Information quality and availability significantly influence business practices and culture; they are fundamental factors in the path that health care takes in the future (see Chapter 1). Decisions about collecting and using information depend on management attitudes and vision, on tradition and leadership style, and on goals and business values. The enhanced ability to spread "information currency" around means that decision making can be decentralized, operational controls relaxed, and accountability dispersed in new ways. The new capabilities challenge traditional ideas about enterprise roles and structure, from the organization chart to bricks and mortar. The appearance of telemedicine, the distribution of medical advice and test results electronically, and interactive patient-physician exchanges over the Internet are examples.

Traditional Structure

The traditional way of picturing enterprise structure involves hierarchy, with fixed relationships that reflect relative responsibility and power. Organization charts have been flipped every which way by business pundits, with customers at the top, the bottom, the center, and the periphery, but they still imply stratification. There has been recent conjecture about the potential of freely flowing information to flatten such hierarchies.[1] This "technocentric" prediction is a reasonable view theoretically, but it may not be optimal from a human standpoint, because such flattening is likely to be unacceptable to everyone inside the enterprise except the denizens of the bottom row.

Other methods of describing organization structure have been developed to address current business complexities, one example of which is the *organization matrix.* This convention maps roles and responsibilities rather than merely indicating who gets to tell whom what to do, and it displays those who are responsible for vertical functions as well as those who are in charge of horizontal (cross-functional) areas. For example, one individual may be responsible for marketing (vertical), but another is responsible for publications and communications across all functions including marketing (horizontal)— hence a matrix. *(Something within what or from which something else originates, develops or takes form)*

Students of organization structure have compared enterprises to ecological systems and sociologic communities and considered models ranging from psychological mirroring to hardened technology; they have typified them by bureaucracies of various kinds (simple, machine, professional, ad hoc, divisionalized) and arranged them in political archetypes ranging from monarchy to federalism.[2-4]

In the information age, a more useful structural framework would place emphasis on the role of information in the conduct of business, focus on organization integration through information systems, and minimize hierarchy. It would promote the idea of variable centers of influence, anticipate real-time control of operations, emphasize shifts of responsibility between functional areas, enhance responsiveness to fluctuating internal and external conditions, and suggest evolution paths to more efficient processes. It would accentuate the role of information in growth, specialization, cooperation, and differentiation and would be more fluid in nature than the fixed engineering models that have been defined in the past.

The structural model I believe encompasses these desirable characteristics is a reflection of life processes, and the "bio-enterprise" framework that follows is based on fundamental biological principles. The ideas for the bio-enterprise framework are based on experience with clinical information systems in a large, geographically dispersed, integrated health maintenance organization and on observations of the benefits of information technology in successful companies referred to as "the electronic elite."[5] They are particularly useful in understanding the potential impacts of information on care delivery structures, be they staff-model HMOs, physician managed care organizations, hospital services, preferred provider organizations, or fee-for-service private practices.

In the "Introduction" at the beginning of this book, I suggested that working with modern business components is more like manipulating water than ice. Whereas ice can be arranged in a hierarchy (at least for a little while), with the blocks at the top, the cubes in the middle, and the shavings at the bottom, working with water requires very different tools and techniques. Because all living creatures on earth depend on and are primarily composed of water, their structure and modes of operation are quite instructive.

The 'Bio-Enterprise' Framework

The bio-enterprise framework draws analogies between corporation structures and four basic life-forms: _protozoa_ (single cell), _sponge_ (multi-cellular), _simple animal_, and _complex animal_. The cell is the basic unit of plant and animal life that is capable of reproducing and living independently, given appropriate environmental conditions. More than one cell living with another creates a multicellular organism, and, as the multicellular organisms get more complex and larger, they are referred to as plants if they make their food out of sunlight (photosynthesis) or as animals if they ingest things as nutrients. Simple animals have been a bit arbitrarily defined in this metaphor as multicellular organisms without a heart and blood vessels (circulatory system). The distinction between simple and complex animals (those with circulatory systems) is for purposes of illustration only; you will see why a little later.

There are some very important general principles to consider before delving into structural models. Basic life mechanisms _(metabolism)_ are essentially the same across the spectrum of these forms. The maintenance of life depends on the ability of a living unit, whether one cell or many, to maintain internal operating conditions within a certain range, even though the outside world may change. What distinguishes one form from another, and, comparatively, one organization structure from another, is the quality of communication and cooperation between units via information.

It is a law of physics that, in any equilibrium situation, all processes will tend toward disorder and randomness. Because living processes require order and stability to exist, energy must be obtained and work performed by them in order to oppose this force and maintain life. The process of maintaining stability is called _homeostasis_, and it can be compared to the ability of an enterprise to remain financially sound. Resources are expended to produce items or services that have the effect of sustaining the organization in a specific market environment. How much resources are spent, how available raw nutrients are, how reliable the internal environment is, how stable the external world remains, and precisely how work is performed all determine survival in a way that is quite analogous to metabolic life processes. Homeostasis can be thought of as the ultimate state of cost-efficiency.

Using life form analogies encourages thinking about organizations in light of their size, complexity, integration, cooperation, interdependence, and ability to adapt to change. Because maintenance of life, regardless of structure, depends on the precise execution of millions of metabolic pathways carried out by separate but highly interdependent cellular entities, the initial lesson for all enterprises is that balanced cooperative individual performance, not power or stature, are the essential elements of successful function.

Protozoan

The maintenance of life depends on the ability of a living unit, whether one cell or many, to maintain internal operating conditions within a certain range, even though the outside world may change.

The first model is named after single-celled organisms called protozoans, and it represents the structure of many small businesses, as well as of departments in larger enterprises. Protozoans are solitary organisms that depend almost exclusively on their nucleus for direction and survival. The nucleus is responsible for initiating reproduction, passing on genetic material to progeny, and directing cellular activities. It has a controlling role in this model, directing the creation of substances and cell work units (called organelles). There is some juice around the nucleus, called cytoplasm, within which the organelles carry out millions of cellular processes independently of the nucleus, once they have gotten the nuclear message. In business, the central mission similarly directs work activities, but independent operational realization of core goals by nonnuclear entities is critical for enterprise sustenance. Finally, there is a thin cell membrane around the cytoplasm that separates the organism from the outside world and regulates the movement of water and chemicals between the cytoplasm and the surrounding environment.

A key here is that protozoans, as unicellular animals, are completely surrounded by the environment and therefore focus entirely on stability within their isolated structure; they are "generalists" that metabolize and divide but do not specialize. These creatures are not simple in a biochemical sense, but structurally they are relatively "dumbed down." They do sense elements of their environment in a rudimentary way by means of special recognition receptors that are embedded in their surrounding cell membrane, but communication with other organisms, alike or not, is unnecessary. In fact, most protozoans view each other as little more than food chain items. General operating procedures for protozoans are similar to the determinants of success in old-style, traditional, militaristic businesses: Search, ingest, destroy, digest, and split (not necessarily in that order).

Individuals, departments, and entire companies can be observed that exhibit predominately protozoan characteristics. "Nuclear" CEOs or department chiefs emphatically proclaim a full awareness of all information needed to get a job done and how to obtain it. They insist on strict control of internal surroundings and communications, profess no need to receive data from other departments, and are likely to believe that their operations are so streamlined and efficient that information other than what they are accustomed to will only confuse things and "gum up the works." They command the unit and are generally autocratic and fiercely purposeful; doctors may be the ultimate protozoans.

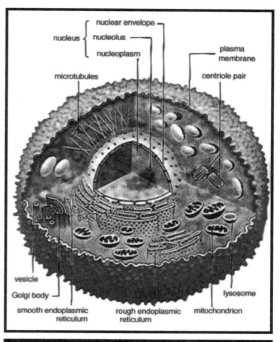

Three dimensional sketch of a typical animal cell showing the nucleus and other organelles. (From: The Unity and Diversity of Life, 6th edition)

The problem for single-celled organisms, however, is size. They are giants when barely visible to the unaided human eye. This is because the volume of the cell increases more quickly than does its surface area.

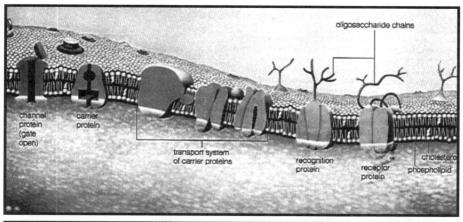

Drawing of the membrane that separates the cytoplasm (inside of the cell) from the environment. Note the protein receptors that function in recognition and regulation of trans-membrane processes. (From: The Unity and Diversity of Life, 6th edition)

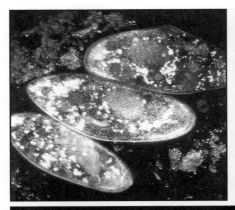
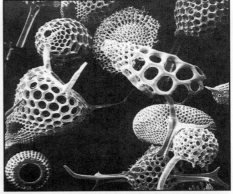

Light microscopic images protozoans, Paramecium and a set of radiolarian 'skeletons'.
(From: Life on Earth)

Therefore, a threshold is reached at which the metabolic needs of the cytoplasm outstrip the abilities of the cell membrane to balance and regulate inner and outer activities; metabolic processes become inefficient, and, no matter how much control is exerted by the nucleus, the cell begins to fail.

Some monolithic companies have tried to maintain the protozoan model as their size increased to unnatural proportions. Increasing nuclear control, kicking cytoplasm organelles around, and demanding more "work" has not altered the fact that, above a threshold size, the entire structure needs to change, or some massive downsizing (excuse me, right-sizing) needs to be undertaken to recover homeostasis.[6] This model is in no way substandard and does not imply poor quality. It may be immaculately appropriate. Size may become an issue and vulnerability to minor environmental stress a concern, but at least there is no need for an expensive high-maintenance information system. Besides, how can one argue with a 1,200 million year track record? There are more than 10,000 known species of protozoans, with varying methods for gathering nutrients (resource management), moving around (exploring the market), reproducing (franchising), and protecting themselves from environmental risks (patents, lawyers). They constitute more than half of the earth's biomass.

At some point, a set of "toughminded," innovative protozoans must have become dissatisfied with metabolically imposed growth restrictions, or perhaps they discovered survival benefits that accrued to colonial living fortuitously, and a fundamental change from the unicellular organism to the multicellular organism transpired. This is exemplified by Volvox, unicellular green algae that stick together in groups of up 50,000 to form a hollow sphere. Each organism has a flagellum that it beats to generate motion. Flagella are tail-like modifications of the cell membrane that function as undulating propellers to create movement; a lot of them in groupings on a cell are called cilia. Once stuck together, however, Volvox communicate with one another in such a way that regional flagella, oriented outward, beat in coordinated unison, carrying the colony in a purposeful direction in the fashion of a rolling ball.

This unification of purpose is facilitated by chemical messages that act locally between adjacent cells and by very fine cytoplasmic bridges between cells. The attachment of a messenger molecule sent from one member to a receptor molecule on the neighbor's membrane induces predictable behavior in the "cell mate." Such messages can be thought of as the ultimate particles of information.

This is a splendid real-life example of the concept of business synergy and of win-win philosophy. A solution is apparent that is good for all and beneficial beyond the sum of the Volvox. There isn't a boss in this model, just a group of motivated individuals flailing together. Each individual is responsible for itself, but, like humans, they seem to enjoy community.

Some monolithic companies have tried to maintain the protozoan model as their size increased to unnatural proportions.

Cooperation and communication in the colony also allow for specialization, in that some few lucky cells are signaled to become reproductive, their raison d'être no longer being motion or nutrient gathering but production of progeny. The special cells divide to form "daughter" colonies inside the sphere and, at a precise time, release different information messages to the mother colony cells, causing them to momentarily unstick from each other in a region to allow birth.

Suddenly, within the multi-celled organism, cooperation and communication allow growth and diversity to appear. Recall from your reading of empowerment, personal development, and leadership literature the number of times that growth has been a key element. From Covey[4] to Robbins[7] to Batten,[8] to the James,[1,5] growth is fundamental to achievement and business performance. Certainly one can grow in "size" or "depth" or "complexity" or "values" or "spirit"; the point is that great organizations will find a way to grow, regardless of external limits.[9] Imagine the response of a traditional corporation to the

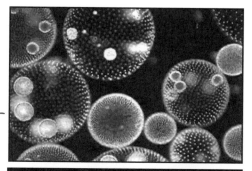

Light microscope view of several Volvox colonies. Note the daughter colonies within the "motherships". (From: The Unity and Diversity of Life, 6th edition)

---

proposal of a small department to take on all the sexual reproduction for the company. Yet exactly this kind of "no rules" thinking (well, maybe not exactly) defines leading companies today.

The second lesson for organizations from this model is that moving from solitary-style business operations (solo fee-for-service practice, for example) to larger diversified enterprise structures (IPA, HMO, PPO) or from one-on-one patient-doctor disease management to team-population based health care interventions requires new methods for communicating, reacting, and cooperating. It is wise to bear in mind that in true multicellular organisms such as Volvox, in contradistinction to merely colonial unicellular organisms living together, the benefits of size, diversity, and increased capability carry some risk in that the organisms can no longer live in isolation. The organism dies if the colony is disrupted.

Sponge

Sponges are slightly more complex than Volvox, and the second model of organizational structure is based on them. They have a double layer of cells that form a more intricate and complicated structure than a hollow sphere. There is an inner surface that is lined with flagellated cells (pointing inward), an outer layer of flattened non-flagellated cells, and in-between these layers a semi-fluid layer of material that contains a few unique ameboid cells and some hard silica spicules that support the structure like a skeleton. There are minuscule holes, called pores, at regular intervals in the layered sheets of the sponge, and, as the flagellated cells of the inner lining beat in unison, they draw water and nutrients from the surrounding water through the pores to the inside, where collars of the inner lining cells can filter, trap, and ingest food particles. (The water drawn in through the pores is expelled through a single larger "vent" in the organism.) Nutrients absorbed by the flagellated cells are partially used and then passed to the middle layer ameba cells, which further

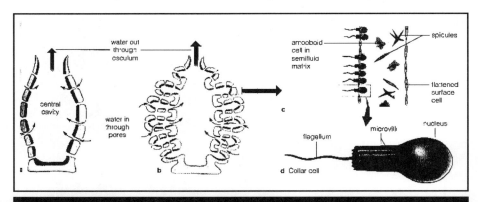

A diagram of the components of a multicellular organism, the sponge. Note the beauty of cooperative function. (From: The Unity and Diversity of Life, 6th edition)

digest and store them. The ameboid cells further distribute nutrients to the outer lining cells and also manufacture the supporting spicules and goo within the central layer. Sometimes the ameboid cells secrete little shells around themselves rather than spicules; this is important to you only because the shells, spicules, and hardened goo are what you use to wash your back in the shower.

A great advance in specialization and cooperation is exemplified by the sponge. Grouped units have well-defined tasks for the maintenance of form, function, and equilibrium. The flagellated cells move water, trap and ingest food, and pass on nutrients, while the outer lining cells protect the organism from environmental hazards and the central layer cells support their sandwiching compatriots. Aggregations of cooperating individuals with unique strengths and purposes contribute to cohesive, holistic growth and survival.

> The activities of more sophisticated cooperative coordinated multi-cellular organisms are enabled by the actions of chemical messages (the communication of information) and the sharing of resources between cells. Sharing information promotes growth and success.

The sponge pristinely illustrates a number of characteristics pointed out by Covey[4] as parts of what he calls the Principle Centered Leadership Paradigm (PCL)—particularly the holistic characteristic, wherein different work-styles and skills are aligned and cohesive, and the ecological characteristic, meaning initiatives in one area (food capture) effect other areas within the greater environment. Covey points out streams or operational environments inside an organization that need to be monitored to keep conditions aligned with external realities. The sponge actually creates a stream of its own with its internal flagella to feed all of its components.

The activities of more sophisticated cooperative coordinated multi-cellular organisms are enabled by the actions of chemical messages (the communication of information) and the sharing of resources between cells. Sharing information promotes growth and success.

Extension of the sponge model to business involves adaptive but limited sharing of information between organization departments, with maintenance of a strong sense of departmental autonomy, individuation, and focused purpose. Each department knows how to gather resources and respond to messages using its specific tools and techniques as a group. It may pass on certain information or resources to other departments, in the same way that the flagellated cells pass material to the spicule builders, who share resources with the protective lining cells.

The perception of the departments is that they function as cohesive units with relatively singular purposes, responding most acutely to information in their local internal environment. The sense is that, if each subculture does its job and passes on occasional resources and information to adjacent sections, they can all survive. (What happens to the sponge three inches away from a particular cell locus is relatively unimportant to the total structure.)

This is a classic example of leveraging strengths in a diverse operation; the outer lining cells are not expected to move current and the flagellated cells are not asked to build spicules. Each unit knows what it does best, but only through information communication does the entire organism thrive.

The activities of more sophisticated cooperative coordinated multi-cellular organisms are enabled by the actions of chemical messages (the communication of information) and the sharing of resources between cells. Sharing information promotes growth and success.

To ingrain the *importance* of information in this model, it is interesting to consider the "sieve test" as an intellectual exercise to assess the quality and effectiveness of purposeful communication within an enterprise. The sieve test is based on the fact that, if one takes a sponge (or even two) and gently squeezes it through a sieve such that component cells are separated from one another and dispersed in sea water, they will spontaneously reconstruct themselves into a new sponge. Each cell, regardless of initial parentage, knows its role and place in a larger organism by virtue of molecular recognition and messaging, which are determined innately by the genetic material of each cell. (I have received permission to perform the sieve test in a large computer corporation, but I have preferred to first observe the effects of hostile mergers and downsizing in the wild before experimenting further.)

The lesson here for enterprises is that the greater the degree and sophistication of information and resource sharing the greater are the opportunities for specialization, adaptability and successful redesign.

Simple Animal

Simple animal is an unfair label for the third, more complex structure, in which multicellular organisms coalesce their specialized cells into *tissues*. Tissues are groups of cells and intercellular substances that function in concert to perform a common task; they can be further arranged into organs and organ systems. It is appropriate to wonder where to draw the line here, because the sponge lining cells seem to fit the tissue definition. The distinction is difficult and imprecise, so suffice it to say it is a matter of degree. The point is that the amount of complexity, interdependency, specialization of function, coordination, and organism information sharing reaches a new plane in the simple animal.

The simplest of simple animals are the jellyfish, which are actually quite complicated. They have nerves, simple muscles, poisonous stinging harpoons, eggs, and sperm. They also exhibit transitional forms of staged development, starting out as babies attached by a stalk to something solid and developing in adulthood into their more familiar floating umbrella shaped form. This "staged developmental" element illustrates another characteristic of the PCL management paradigm: sequential ordered processes of business growth and transformation. Sea anemones are also in this group. If you squeeze these organisms through a sieve you get a gross lifeless mess, the lesson being that greater complexity and specialization does have some drawbacks.

Coral, which are also simple animals, offer one of the earliest biological examples of the use of *consultants*. Over their 600 million year engagement with the coral, consultants have taken the form of algae (single-celled plants, for simplicity sake), which use photosynthesis to make nutrients for themselves out of solar energy. They dwell safely within the protective bodies of the coral, and, as they photosynthesize, they absorb carbon dioxide from the water, which provides a concentrated local base of organic substance necessary for the coral to build its protective shell. (The shells, or skeletons, of coral comprise the great sea reefs.) The algae also liberate oxygen during photosynthesis, which the coral cells require to "breathe." This is a wonderful example of a critical element in today's successful corporate environment. (No, not consultants.) *Symbiosis*—the cooperation of different types of organisms in a mutually beneficial relationship. The algae would be a nourishing morsel indeed if the coral cell nucleus was destroy-and-ingest-oriented. The secret of success on the part of the consultants in this case is the relentless recommendation to locate the organization in proximity to sunlight. (It is admittedly easier to be a valued consultant if business disengagement means that the client will have a hard time breathing.)

The most critical element of the simple animal model is the presence of a network of nerve cells that thread through the other tissues, transmitting sensory information and coordinating responses to stimuli. The neural network sends messages to contractile tissues to create motion, to feeding structures to ingest and digest food, and to reproductive centers to facilitate mating and the production of offspring. In many simple animals, the nerve cells further coalesce into a central nerve center, or brain, which maintains a network of interconnections to peripheral structures to monitor processes and to transmit impulses that control operations

Although exceedingly more complex than the protozoan or the sponge, tissues and organs of the simple animal have the same goal: homeostasis—maintenance of a stable internal environment. Each cell unit engages in basic work (metabolism) to ensure its survival, but, at the same time, cells of the tissues or organs perform specialized functions that contribute to survival of the entire creature. This means that, through coordinated collaboration and cellular information communication, separate but integrated structures all work to promote a stable environment for each individual cell.

Maintenance of equilibrium in the simple animal system requires *sensory receptors*, which monitor the environments (internal and external), *integrators* (the brain), which receive and process information and initiate responses to sensory stimuli, and *effectors*, which communicate the brain messages to the relevant organs or tissues. Coordination by the neural network allows remote elements of the structure to influence each other without the need for proximity messaging, thereby facilitating even greater specialization of units, greater efficiency, and directed contributions to organism stability.

> *The most critical element of the simple animal model is the presence of a network of nerve cells that thread through the other tissues, transmitting sensory information and coordinating responses to stimuli.*

This model is analogous to more highly integrated businesses, wherein information is shared over a communication network between departments in a directed fashion, based largely on executive decisions made in the central control center. From a technical computing viewpoint, one might see this as a "network-centric" model of sorts. An example of this method of function might be when materials management senses a sudden decline in critical raw materials, which it communicates to the executive team by voice mail. Managers integrate the information (analyze the situation) and respond by sending pertinent messages to operations, which responsively shift resource usage and begin accessing stored supplies. Similar messages are sent to research, stimulating investigation of alternatives to the scarce resource. Much of this communication can occur electronically over a network, regardless of geographic remoteness.

The presence of brains in organisms (and occasionally in organizations) raises issues around the degree to which the holistic structure must rely on the brain. The control center cannot possibly be responsible for directing every process of the operation (micromanagement); it may influence uniform flagellar motion to move an organism out of a threatening environment, but it cannot be directly responsible for each cell's rhythm. It cannot singly determine all communication messages, standardize all operations, or direct everything that should be sensed or performed by each unit regardless of specialization. Rather, the brain and its extensions must act as coordinators that orchestrate cooperative autonomous functions and must augment survival probability by virtue of its integration capabilities.

The amount of control exerted by the brain's information network, and its relative influence over the autonomy of individuals and departments, is largely determined by leadership style and politics in an enterprise and by the degree of sophistication of its network infrastructure. Regardless of the degree of central control, information communication in simple animals depends on a combination of messages (within the cell, locally between cells, and over neural networks) that have the characteristics of "information" (see chapter 5). The messages must be timely, complete, accurate, relevant, clear, and comprehensible. Messages, in whatever form they are delivered, must be understood; they must occur in standard, reliable recognizable ways. The response to the message may vary, depending on the type of respondent, but commonality of the medium for information communication must be present.

In fact, the chemical information in biological systems provides a very easy way to conceptualize what information really is. The information molecule is three dimensional, and it must fit precisely into the membrane receptor, like a puzzle piece, to induce a desired action. The molecule must be complete and precisely shaped (validity), uncomplicated by irrelevant substances (conciseness and clarity) to be recognized and bound to its receptor. If it is delivered at an inappropriate time (timeliness) or if there is no receptor (relevancy), it will be ineffective in communicating.

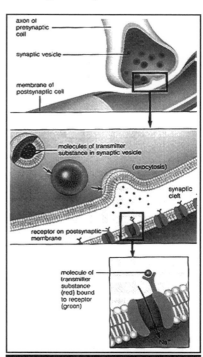

In the case of nerve-conducted messages to tissues, an electrical impulse is transmitted over the cell membrane to the nerve ending, which responds by releasing one of several types of molecular substances called *neurotransmitters*. These chemicals act in a fashion similar to local messaging, in that they attach to receptors on the tissue being informed, causing it to respond in a specific manner. Some tissues receive such messages on a constant basis but take action on the basis of relative concentrations of receptor saturation; others sense the balance of different types of neurotransmitters that are released. The nerve must give a consistent reliable set of messages and speak a "standard language" to the responding tissue, and the sensor (be it sight, touch,

Drawing of the general mechanism of action of neurotransmission at chemical synapses between nerve cells, wherein information flows from one nerve cell to another via chemical messages released in response to neural excitation. (From: The Unity and Diversity of Life, 6th edition)

temperature, sound, etc.) must be able to translate the stimulus into language that the nerve can communicate to the brain.

In biological systems, reactions to information can be categorized into *feedback loops*. In a negative feedback loop, some change in the environment (internal or external) occurs, is sensed by a receptor and is sent to the integrator. The integrator sends a response to an effector, which initiates activity to diminish, dampen, or decrease the intensity of the initial stimulus. Positive feedback is a similar process, but, in this case, the effector works to increase the intensity or magnitude of the change that was initially perceived. In this fashion, the internal environment is kept on an even keel with external stressors and monitored internal metabolic processes, and homeostasis is maintained.

The presence of brains in organisms (and occasionally in organizations) raises issues around the degree to which the holistic structure must rely on the brain.

If there is any single area to concentrate on in evaluating the processes and information flow in an enterprise, it is on this concept of feedback responsiveness, often referred to as workflow. This is really the key to adjusting to conditions on a moment-to-moment basis, a fundamental element of balance.[10] Feedback is key to empowering motivated workers to make decisions rapidly and appropriately and to change their behavior and decisions as conditions vary. It allows adaptation without the anxiety of abandoning an ingrained rule, insulting someone's ego, or risking punishment for having made a potentially wrong move. A splendid concise discussion of feedback variables in systems can be found in the logic of failure.

Using information to effect alterations in a chain or cycle of events is intuitive, but surprisingly few traditional companies have developed high-level capabilities in this area. The more batch reporting, central control, and bureaucratic rules are in place to govern activities, the less likely it is that feedback mechanisms are adequate. No decision is right in perpetuity, so honoring and rewarding flexibility and exploiting the power of feedback is very important. This is a key element of moving from solid (rules) to liquid (judgment) methods of working.

The lesson here is that a higher level of integration, diversity, and capability can be attained (in this case through networks) if communication of meaningful information between subcultures and systems can be carried out. Common, recognizable messages, message formats, communication rules, and mechanical compatibility are called "standards" in the information system world; without standards, integration is nearly impossible. This explains why much attention is being focused presently on the development of common standard clinical terminology for documenting medical activity, which in turn allows medical outcome evaluation; advancement of evidence-based practices; and incorporation of system-based, real-time, automatic decision support (feedback) for medical decision makers.[11]

There is significant evidence that less control and more information-enabled interdependence, in a culture of trust, cooperation, and self-reliance, is a very healthy adaptation.[5]

Complex Animal

Before describing the characteristic information capabilities of complex animals, it is prudent to review a few key items. Individual cells have the means of responding to changes in their environment by virtue of cell membrane receptors that sense specific chemicals or conditions. This allows the protozoan to govern homeostasis, to recognize and ingest food, and to move away from certain toxins.

In colonial protozoans and sponges, there are "signaling" molecules that act as information messengers between local cells; similar messaging exists between tissue cells that function together in animals. The simple animal model brings the nervous system (sensor, integrator, effector) into play as a conductor of information to modulate homeostasis via the effects of neurotransmitters on the receptive tissues.

The complex animal model, for purposes of this exercise, is one that is extremely well integrated, very complex, and enormously information-dependent. The brain and network elements are highly developed and retain critical importance, but additional subsets of communication and response exist that further enhance diversity and adaptability of the organism.

In complex animals, there are billions of cells organized into tissues and organs, each one of which may respond as a unit to a variety of molecular messages. The ultimate in integration, and an analogue of freely flowing information in a business, is regulation of these billions of cellular units by signal molecules called *hormones*. Hormones are chemicals that are released into the blood and diffused into the fluids that bathe the cells of the animal. These chemicals stimulate responses in any cells that have receptors for them; only the cells that have the receptors, called "target cells," respond. The successful use of hormones depends on a circulatory system, the ultimate communication medium, wherein virtually every integrated structural member is bathed in connectivity. A circulation system allows use of information on the basis of the receptiveness, needs, and local conditions of each cell unit.

There is enormous adaptability and specialization of structure and function possible in this model, which allows for exploitation of previously forbidding niches and for the development of marvelous variation. As with other biological messaging, individual cell or tissue responses are predictable, modulated through feedback mechanisms, and holistically oriented. Hormones may effect all of the cells of an organism or only those of a specific organ system, depending on the messages and the targets. They may act directly or may influence other hormone-producing cells to release different substances that engender an effect indirectly.

The response to hormones is often of a more global character, such as induction of growth, promotion of sexual maturation, influence of blood nutrient availability, regulation of wake-sleep cycles, invocation of life-preserving flight or fight reactions, protection of an organism from infection or injury, regulation of the timing of physiologic functions, or alteration of metabolic processes in every cellular unit. (They can also be quite specific, as with the chemical message that causes the gall bladder to contract in response to a fatty meal in the stomach.)

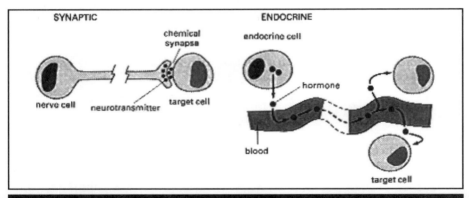

Drawing of two means of signaling by secreted molecules, synaptic (neurotransmission and endocrine (hormonal). (From: Molecular Biology of the Cell, Third Edition)

Hormones are manufactured by cells in *glands of the endocrine* system, which release them in response to sensors they possess to monitor conditions. In addition to these sensors, the endocrine system is also subject to regulation by the nervous system; some nerves actually produce hormones rather than neurotransmitters. There is a subtle interactive blending, or interface, between the two complex but distinguishable information regulation mechanisms.

In business, hormones represent free-flowing data elements released by units in response to changing internal or external conditions for use as information by any individuals or departments who are receptive. In everyday life, an analogy here might be be the radio/television waves in which all of us are emerged constantly, responding only to those we choose to tune into. The signals can have profound effects throughout the entire enterprise, or can stimulate local actions in a subculture. In health care, the complex animal model explains how care practices can shift from isolated doctor-centered models to integrated clinical team health management approaches via flowing information. It also presages a transition from one-on-one treatment models to population-based care and group disease interventions. The idea that patients might someday be "bathed" in relevant health information rather than restricted to sequential interactions with a care provider or system seems quite plausible in light of this model.

The hormonal information system in complex animals allows the brain to monitor and influence corporal functions, but with a relative relaxation of vigilant monitoring and controlling; it allows more time for thinking. System autonomy, cooperation, and interdependence are augmented; routine, less strategic operations seem to look out for themselves, and the brain can focus on vision, planning, guidance, and more volitional functions.

In humans, the pinnacle of complex animals (since we get to make the definitions and describe the science), there is the distinguishing characteristic of the ability to plan. Leadership in the pure modern sense means setting course, inspiring corporeal loyalty, changing, growing, adapting, and adjusting, with foresight!

Common, recognizable messages, message formats, communication rules, and mechanical compatibility are called "standards" in the information system world; without standards, integration is nearly impossible.

The complex animal metaphor also represents the transformation being achieved in mature information age enterprises. The development of systems that enhance information flow has allowed evolution of businesses in the direction of greater integration, complexity, diversity, autonomy, and interdependence.

Integration

Information system integration bears a bit more scrutiny in light of the bio-enterprise framework. In business, integration means that information systems communicate with one another in a meaningful way, allowing users to access uniform programs to input information to or to obtain information from disparate systems on various platforms with vastly different core functions. The connection of systems is very hard to achieve (which is why they are often referred to as "legacy" systems), but it is critical for uniting organization structure. This kind of integration requires standards for data communication between systems that are adhered to, as well as commonalty of data definition, transmission, interpretation, and presentation. In most instances, this means that a common terminology or lexicon must be present and that conventions for sharing the uniform data are adhered to.

This is quite analogous to the neurotransmitter/hormone concept, in which messages are delivered via standard signals but the cardiovascular system responds differently from the gastrointestinal system, which responds differently from the cartilage cells in the growth plates of bones. Cooperative function mandates communication standards and easy data translation ("integration engines," interface standards, and "open architecture blueprints" are evolving to allow this, but the efforts are still very expensive).

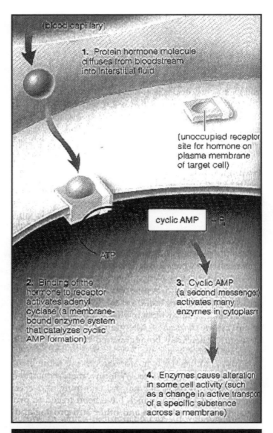

(blood capillary)

1. Protein hormone molecule diffuses from bloodstream into interstitial fluid

(unoccupied receptor site for hormone on plasma membrane of target cell)

cyclic AMP + P

ATP

2. Binding of the hormone to receptor activates adenyl cyclase (a membrane-bound enzyme system that catalyzes cyclic AMP formation)

3. Cyclic AMP (a second messenger) activates many enzymes in cytoplasm

4. Enzymes cause alteration in some cell activity (such as a change in active transport of a specific substance across a membrane)

Drawing of the method oaction of protein hormones when they bind specifically to surface receptors on target cells. (From: The Unity and Diversity of Life, 6th edition)

As integration is achieved between information systems in an enterprise, legacy system experts, information technologists, and operations managers will face the new challenge of constant interactions and shared decision making, because what used to be relatively independent changes in previously isolated areas will now have impacts on everyone else in the organization. Even simple equipment upgrades or software version releases can affect the entire network or can corrupt databases or interfaces, so either independence gives way to cooperation or everything collapses. A change control board, or something like it, should be convened to evaluate and authorize even minor changes to linked systems. In fact, such a coordinating body is important in evaluating new system acquisitions or development as well, to be sure that silo applications that can't be integrated or that break operation functions elsewhere don't spring up unintentionally.

There are three terms related to integration that can cause great problems if confused with it. One is convergence, when it implies that systems or technology should *converge* to a single platform solution. Used in this fashion, convergence means "pick an organ and everyone use it." This is very distinct from integration, which does not require an entire organism to be, for instance, a liver.

Ideally, convergence signals a move toward shared data models, common terminology, unified coding schemes, and standard communication protocols so that information can be shared, compared, and understood, regardless of where, how, or on what platform it is derived. The analogy in biology is the use of common neurotransmitters and messaging molecules to coordinate processes. (The term as it is used here is distinct from the phenomenon of industry convergence, which describes the situation in which what used to be separate entities (telephone services, computing, broadcasting, entertainment, education, publishing, etc.) are coalescing into conglomerate media enterprises.)[12]

Even simple equipment upgrades or software version releases can affect the entire network or can corrupt databases or interfaces, so either independence gives way to cooperation or everything collapses.

The second, and a closely related, concept is that of *common systems*, which again suggests that benefits to the whole will accrue if all of the parts use the same system to accomplish their work. The common system approach only works if each individual or department or organization performs the same functions in precisely the same way under the same external pressures and within the same cultural constructs. What may seem like a good idea from a scale and leverage standpoint can actually be maladaptive, trapping units in mediocrity, stifling innovation, and limiting evolution. In fact, common systems are often a myth; even well-conceived identical systems deployed in differing environments remain common for a matter of milliseconds before local information system departments make code changes to suit specific provincial operations needs. What starts as a common system quickly diverges out of the need to maintain local homeostasis. No matter how noble the attempt, forcing information system uniformity on distinct environments, different business practices, or incompatible structural models is usually a costly, short-lived substitute for true integration.

"Convergence" is a good term when referring to data definitions and terminology, and "common" is a good term when referring to communication protocols and information representations, but, beyond this, they can be counter-evolutionary and regressive concepts.

The final "C" of the trio, which is enormously vogue today, is "componentization." Heralded with the same optimism and suggested simplicity that surrounded the introduction of client server architecture a decade ago, it posits that object-related technology will allow development of highly integrated information systems with interchangeable functional components. This notion is quite seductive, but the problem is that the majority of information systems (particularly clinical information systems) are not of the same species or genus (or even kingdom), and, by the time an ideal "componentized," truly integrated beast is built, capable of disassembly and rapid incorporation into another complementary beast, technology will undoubtedly be offering a next solution, leaving behind what is little more than a hard-won but outmoded "common system."

Componentization (formerly sometimes referred to as modularity, a *tool-based solution*) is very promising, but, if one delays integration efforts along the lines of data structure, vocabulary, and communication standards while waiting for a component solution, the only effects to accrue will be those of age and infirmity (or the distasteful alternative).

Anything Else?

The bio-enterprise framework is meant to assist in understanding the role of information systems in an enterprise; as with all analogies, it should be used for illumination, not for support. There is no simple survey, check list, or recipe for classification, and the metaphor should not be taken to extremes. In fact, most businesses have some segments that function like single cells and others that are more akin to the complex animal. The base concepts, not the details, are what matter.

Ideally, convergence signals a move toward shared data models, common terminology, unified coding schemes, and standard communication protocols so that information can be shared, compared, and understood, regardless of where, how, or on what platform it is derived.

These categories do not imply inherent value; the desire may be to have an organization be the complex animal type because it seems more highly evolved and more impressive in its diversity and ingenuity, but realize that the lowly protozoan and sponge are among the world's most successful life forms. Also realize that anything that is alive can die if the environment changes in an extreme way or if internal processes fail to maintain stability. For a protozoan, an extreme change might be a couple of degrees of temperature in the surroundings or some chlorine in the water, whereas generally greater variances can be tolerated by more complex animals.

Whether an enterprise structure is conceptualized as protozoan, sponge, or simple/complex animal (or some combination), it comprises humans with individual brains. In humans, the brain occasionally thinks, but it always generates emotions, which can influence thoughts, decisions, and responses. This emotional factor throws politics and psychology into the biological mix, regardless of the enterprise structure.

The protozoan, sponge, and simple and complex animal models can all be successful as long as environmental alterations do not exceed their relative abilities to adjust and adapt. The protozoan will never pole vault, but the complex animal will never split in two. An advanced information system is never the only thing needed for success. Be wary of technocratic utopians who suggest otherwise.[3] Nowhere in nature, as far as I know, is there a viable entity that comprises only messages, or solely nerves. Hormones in isolation are inanimate.

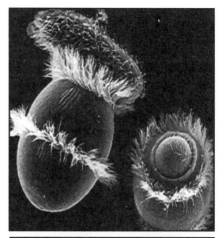

Scanning electron micrograph of a big-mouthed ciliated protozoan (Didinium) engaging in some nutritional activity involving a paramecium. (From: The Unity and Diversity of Life, 6th edition)

Many aspects of business, medicine, information systems, and life vicissitudes can be cast in an amusing light; maintaining emotional balance is an important element of clear thinking as evolution proceeds. Just about the time beating protozoan (paramecium) cilia are coordinated with a new nuclear messaging system that allows movement at a speed of ten times its body length per second (about 40 miles per hour for humans), a big didinium that has focused on developing a huge coordinated feeding structure, merges with it in a less than auspicious fashion. Right after a Volvox joins forces with its comrades to form a sphere of safety (with a local messaging network), coordinating motion, a sponge sucks it through a pore, traps it in a collar, and passes its partially digested carcass to the spicule builders. Even as this is happening, a sea urchin (simple animal) is devouring the sponge's outer lining cells, which tasty treat it detected via its distributed nervous system (despite the fact that it doesn't have a brain). Fully nourished and happy in its niche, the echinoderm is plucked from the reef by a young human entrepreneur, whose heart races with excitement from the release of

Componentization (formerly sometimes referred to as modularity, a tool-based solution) is very promising, but if one delays integration efforts along the lines of data structure, vocabulary, and communication standards while waiting for a component solution, the only effects to accrue will be those of age and infirmity (or the distasteful alternative).

adrenaline associated with the thought of how much he will be paid for the specimen when he sells it at the aquarium shop back home.

Finally, recognize that growth and evolution occur incrementally, gradually and often painfully, or not at all.[8,13] Patience and time are required to transform from a unicellular animal to a multicellular one, or to learn enough about business practices and enterprise processes to actually implement a helpful information system. The time needed to make the transition can be agonizing, particularly when the external environment appears to be changing rapidly, but bear in mind that hasty mutations and forced adaptations often result in another biologic phenomenon: extinction.

If you are frustrated by the speed with which information systems can be developed and implemented, you might wish to consider the following conjecture about the development of multi-cellularity: "Why was multi-cellularity so slow to evolve? Although the answer cannot be known, it seems likely to be related to the need of a multi-cellular organism for elaborate signal mechanisms that enable its cells to communicate with one another so as to coordinate their behavior for the benefit of the organism as a whole. Intercellular signals, interpreted by complex machinery in the responding cell, allow each cell to determine its position and specialized role in the body.[14]

We speak of the body as a machine, but it is hardly necessary to say that none of the most ingenious machines set up by modern science can for a moment compare with it. The body is a self-building machine; a self-stoking, self-regulating, self-repairing machine. The most marvelous and unique mechanism in the universe.—Sir J. Arthur Thompson, Scottish biologist, 1900.

References

1. James, J. *Thinking in the Future Tense*. New York, N.Y.: Simon and Schuster, 1996.
2. Lewin, K. *Field Theory in Social Science*. New York, N.Y.: Harper and Brothers, 1957.
3. Davenport, T., and others. "Information Politics." *Sloan Management Review* 34(1):53-65, Fall 1992.
4. Covey, S. *Principle-Centered Leadership*. New York, N.Y.: Simon and Schuster, 1992.
5. James, G. *Business Wisdom of the Electronic Elite*. New York, N.Y.: Random House, 1996.
6. Noer, D. *Healing the Wounds: Overcoming the Trauma of Layoffs and Revitalizing Downsized Organizations*. San Francisco, Calif.: Jossey-Bass Publishers, 1995.
7. Robbins, A. *Awaken the Giant Within*. New York, N.Y.: Simon and Schuster, 1992.

8. Batten J. *Tough-Minded Leadership*. New York, N.Y.: Amacom, 1989.
9. Greiner, L. "Evolution and Revolution as Organizations Grow." *Harvard Business Review*, July-Aug. 1972.
10. Dörner, D. *The Logic of Failure,* Reading, Mass.:Addison-Wesley Publishers, 1996, pp. 73-79.
11. Cohn, S., and Chute, C. "Clinical Terminology and Computer-Based Patient Records." JAMIA 68(2):241-73, Feb. 1997.
12. Tapscott, D. *The Digital Economy: Promise and Peril in the Age of Networked Intelligence*. New York, N.Y.: McGraw-Hill, 1996.
13. Arthur, W. "How Fast Is Technology Evolving." *Scientific American* 272(2):105-7, Feb. 1997.
14. Alberts, B., and others. *Molecular Biology of the Cell*.
New York, N.Y.: Garland Publishing, Inc., 1994, p. 721.

Chapter 8

Enterprise Change Management and Information Systems

A living thing is distinguished from a dead thing by the multiplicity of the changes at any moment taking place in it.—Herbert Spencer, English philosopher, 1865.

Implementing a new information system is an intricate and tumultuous process that can magnify *infobia* and foment resistance to becoming a *learning organization*. Companies fail when they underestimate the effort, expense, and expertise necessary to successfully manage the human change that accompanies technology introduction. This is not to trivialize the enormous challenges of creating an enterprise model; understanding the *functional requirements of users*; designing, developing, and testing the *software*; and installing the *platforms and networks* needed to support the new environment, all of which are required to even have something worth changing for.

Add to this the nontechnical impediments to harvesting gains from the painstakingly instituted system, and you may ask: "Why would anyone embark on a task so hard to conceive, difficult to define, arduous to evaluate, strenuous to develop, hazardous to deploy, and exhausting to capitalize on?" Difficult change is undertaken to maintain *homeostasis*; if the environment becomes unfavorable, operations may need to be altered, functions rethought, focus shifted, internal and external conditions reassessed, units integrated, and activities modulated to restore balance. Some have called such processes *reengineering*. In some cases, even gross errors in judgment, well implemented, can be fortuitous. This is really what chance mutations and natural selection are all about.

> Companies fail when they underestimate the effort, expense, and expertise necessary to successfully manage the human change that accompanies technology introduction.

Although this chapter is primarily aimed at managers who are attempting to introduce new systems and create positive change in their companies (and therefore may be of great interest to health care leaders who would like doctors to use computers and change their habits), its principles are also useful for individual clinicians who want a deeper understanding of what keeps them from doing things differently.

The topic of technology-driven change in organizations has received great attention in recent years, and numerous models and approaches have been advanced.[1-3] Most successful approaches involve an understanding of social and behavioral techniques, with attention to vision, respect, involvement, empowerment, teamwork, customer focus, openness to change, and a host of intelligent strategies (from design through implementation).[2] Prior to touching on some of these specific areas, I would like to develop another life science metaphor that will help with visualizing and recalling the most important elements.

The Bio-Transition Framework

Biological systems use energy to maintain the balance between their internal and external physical environments in a process referred to as homeostasis, meaning "standing the same." A classical understanding of energy is not necessary to follow this metaphor. Energy can be conceived of simply as the effort it takes to accomplish work.

Living systems expend energy on processes when it is needed to maintain equilibrium and stability. This balance occurs within an assiduously regulated narrow range; in the absence of this miraculous regulation, everything careens chaotically toward randomness and disorder in accord with the second law of thermodynamics. This law, also called the law of entropy, is what Einstein felt was "the only physical theory of universal content which I am convinced, within the framework of applicability of its basic concepts, will never be overthrown."[4] Life processes, in fact, do not really escape entropy at all, but simply use energy from the surrounding environment to maintain internal order. This results in greater disorder in the external environment to compensate for the increased order (decreased randomness) within the living organism, because the total energy must remain constant. Absent that absorbed energy, however, the internal order cannot be maintained, and universal energy equilibrium is reached, which we call "death." Life opposes, rather than escapes, entropy. Homeostasis can be alternatively thought of as the energy-consuming work of resisting constant universal pressure to go toward lower energy and greater entropy. Some have observed entropy first hand in businesses. Entropy ensues when the "going out of business" sign goes up.

Change and Energy States

Change can be viewed as a move from an initial state to a final state. Energy will need to be put into the transition, and the final state will ultimately have to be beneficial to the total system if the change is to last. This means the end state involves less pain, more pleasure, or less ongoing energy expenditure. It is very important to recognize that, even when the final state is preferable, a certain amount of effort has to be put into making the transition. Natural scientists represent this process in what is called an *energy state diagram* (see figure on page 152). A change can be made to a less preferable state, but, because the natural tendency of events is toward states of lower energy, the less preferable end state is unstable, and a lot of ongoing work will have to be done to keep the end state from regressing.

The amount of energy it takes to make the transition to the final state, the "push" required to achieve the change, is called the activation energy. Activation energy therefore mandates the size of the hill over which we must be pushed to change from one state to another.

Change can be viewed as a move from an initial state to a final state. Energy will need to be put into the transition, and the final state will ultimately have to be beneficial to the total system if the change is to last.

Resistance

If one believes human transition activities need this same push, even when the end state may be more desirable than the current state, one can see that any methods used to decrease the amount of activation energy needed to get over the hill will facilitate the change. (In this sense, the manager's job is to make molehills out of mountains.) This activation energy, or *transition state energy*, has a more familiar name: resistance. Managing the transition state is managing resistance; resistance is normal, necessary, and even critical to maintaining business balance.

Conservation of energy/effort in human behavior is clear: In the absence of external pressures or powerful internal drives to shift responses, humans save energy and maintain the comfort and stability of psychological homeostasis. Our experiences as humans and managers (not mutually exclusive terms, of course) tell us any behavioral change requires energy. Actions and patterns of thinking that are unfamiliar or uncomfortable are not likely to occur spontaneously. Deviations from the accustomed are motivated either by the desire to increase pleasure or by the need to decrease pain. When motivation is high, gratification can be delayed and discomfort endured while laboring toward a desirable end; if motivation is not high, however, or if the new state is perceived as threatening, the status quo remains preferable.

In fact, a business without resistance would consist of unpredictable random changes (chaos), all in the direction of greater entropy. Resistance, or activation energy, is therefore an important leverage point. If transitions and change are managed well, business can thrive and grow, and balance can be maintained. The most sophisticated and elegant change management techniques are those employed by living systems.

In cellular metabolic pathways, substances with an ability to enter into a reaction are called *reactants (or substrates)* before the change and *end products* afterward. Because pathways hand items down an assembly (or disassembly) line of sorts, the end product of one reaction can be the substrate for the next reaction. During each change step, two key items are involved: *enzymes*, which lower activation energy and thereby speed the transition from substrate to product, and energy carriers, which either donate the energy to make things happen or capture the energy released during the change from initial to final state.

Some metabolic pathways break down complex materials (starch to simple sugars, for example), releasing energy from chemical bonds that is captured by uncharged *energy carriers* (usually ADP) for use in other cell processes. The products of the breakdown pathway are of lower energy themselves but are of innate stability similar to or greater than the original, bigger substance. Other cellular pathways assemble smaller molecules

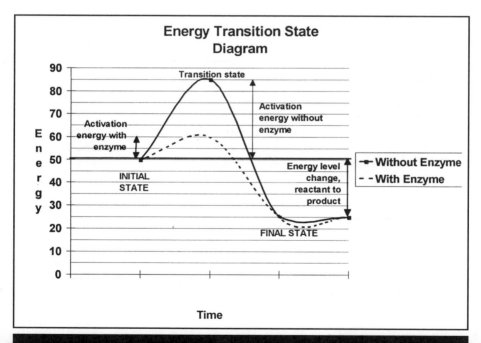

Curves representing the beginning and end energy states of a reaction, and the energy hill (activation energy) necessary for transition to occur. The upper curve shows the amount of energy required without an enzyme facilitator, the lower curve the same reaction with the catalyst. (From: The Unity and Diversity of Life, 6th edition)

into larger, more complex ones, using charged-up energy carriers (usually ATP) to donate energy to the task of combining the reactants, which store the donated energy in their chemical bonds but which are also innately stable (such as with the assembly of complex carbohydrates from simple sugars). In either case, the breakdown or buildup steps require a certain energy input to transform the reactants from an initial state to a final state.

One can think of the reactants as current business entities and processes and the end products as a new way of doing things; the amount of resources spent to create the change will depend on the techniques and individuals used to induce it (change agents/enzymes), and the benefits recovered from the final state will depend on resource capture by *management discipline* (energy carriers).

Catalysts and Benefit Realization

Enzymes are large, complex, folded, three-dimensional protein molecules that enhance the rate at which metabolic reactions occur. They work by lowering the amount of activation energy needed to get to end product (said another way, they decrease the amount of energy needed to get reactants to the hilltop transition state). Four immutable characteristics of enzymes can be compared to business process change management.

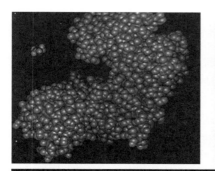 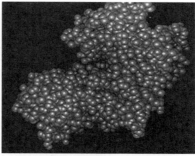

These models show the induced miniscule change an enzyme (hexokinase) undergoes in response to binding with its tiny reactant. The small glucose molecule fits into the active site of the larger enzyme inducing the temporary flexing of the protein around the substrate. (From: The Unity and Diversity of Life, 6th edition)

- *Speed*: Enzymes only speed reactions that could naturaly occur on their own; they do not cause things to happen that could not eventually happen without them. Similarly, one might wish to speed the acceptance and use of computers in an enterprise, but no agent can get the reaction to go if the hardware doesn't exist or the programs aren't compatible with operations.

- *Survival*: Enzymes are not permanently altered or consumed in the reactions they catalyze and can be used repeatedly. In business, when crusaders for change are destroyed during a transition, something has gone terribly wrong; it is natural for the catalyst to survive the change process.

- *Specificity*: Enzymes are very specific and extremely particular about the reactions they catalyze. Because of their folded structure, they have very selective three-dimensional binding or active sites into which their reactants, and only their reactants, can fit. They are, however, slightly flexible, such that binding with their matched substrate causes them to shift shape a little, which provides the molecular bond stress needed to break the reactant down or which brings the two reactants into proximity so that they can bond naturally. Change agents in business transformations are most effective when paired with reactants that are a complementary match. An executive may be perfectly suited to initiate change in other leaders but unable to catalyze front-line behavior changes. The front-line substrates may simply not be the right shape to fit in the executive binding site.

- *Adjusting*: Enzymes can catalyze reactions in two directions; they can put reactants together to make a single entity, or they can take the combined entity apart. What the enzyme does depends on the relative concentrations of reactants and products in the enzyme environment, on complex *feedback loops*, on other cellular molecular messages, and on super-vision by other enzymes. This is important, because in both biology and business, serial changes do not occur in isolation, but rather as a result of multiple change agents, reactants, and products acting in concert.

The incredible multitude of reactions and grinding pathways that are occurring simultaneously in the cell demonstrate that what might appear as chaos is actually beautifully orchestrated cooperation, interdependence, balance, and cohesive autonomy. Homeostasis depends on the ability of organisms to communally adjust and regulate metabolic activities on the basis of supply, demand, and information. Influences on enzymes in metabolic processes may come from the nucleus (department chief) by diffusion, they may arrive via local messaging from an adjacent cell (the division across the hall), they may travel over a neural network (orders from headquarters), or they may be exerted on respondents bathed in hormonal signals (executive team memoranda).

Exactly how the enzyme molecule brings reactants together and provides the stresses to lower the activation energy necessary for them to change into product is fascinating, but it probably doesn't add significant value to this analogy from a business perspective. With just this knowledge,

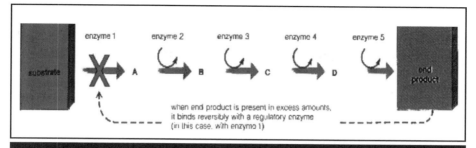

A drawing exemplifying the effect of effect feedback inhibition in a metabolic pathway, keeping things in balance. *(From: The Unity and Diversity of Life, 6th edition)*

however, one can impersonate a cell biologist. Carry around an open Petrie dish, look at the ground, shake your head piteously, and murmur, "I just don't understand what could have gone wrong with this culture." Don't do this without the Petrie dish, though.

Review

Before shifting focus to the core issues of business transition and infobia management in the context of the bio-transition model, a brief summary may be centering. Enzyme catalysts recognize their specific reactants, bring them together in a meaningful way, promote a change, and release product in a controlled fashion based on environmental conditions. When energy is released from the chemical bonds of the reactant as it is changed, it is captured and stored by always attentive energy carriers.

A substance that is a starting reactant for a pathway is acted upon by the first enzyme, which alters it and passes its end product on to the next enzyme in a complex and well-orchestrated series of steps. As the path is negotiated, the energy liberated is harvested at specific points for potential use in other pathways; unharvested energy simply escapes as heat. The balance of energy captured versus energy expended, from end to end, must be favorable for the maintenance of equilibrium between the organism and the outside world.

This kind of pathway assessment was emphasized in the case presentation discussion of Post-Hippocratic Syndrome (see Chapter 1), where considerable weight was placed on looking at the entire set of transitions and costs needed to get from "symptom" to favorable "outcome." As with information system design or change management, balancing energy input and resource utilization with stable favorable end product is the key to creating a homeostatic system.

Bio-Transition, Business, and Infobia Management

There are important lessons to be learned from this biological transition model: Resistance is not only normal, it's the law; it can be equated with the energy of transition or activation energy in the change state diagram. Combine this with an understanding of the core human issues that relate to new information systems, and it becomes clear that managing infobia (see Chapter 6) is critical for lowering the energy of transition.

The biological transition model suggests three major areas to focus on in the drive toward a desired business end state with regard to information systems:

Construct One: Define and Integrate Pathways

Organizational information needs should be determined in the context of enterprise homeostasis, recognizing they are integral to and inseparable from operations. Business pathway components require analysis from end to end. The natural human tendency is to think in simple, short-term, cause-and-effect links, rather than in a more thorough, global, farsighted fashion. Such thinking often leads to short-term success but overall failure, which has led some to observe that our difficulties with complex systems stem from the fact that we have been turned loose on the information age with prehistoric brains.[5]

Enzyme catalysts recognize their specific reactants, bring them together in a meaningful way, promote a change, and release product in a controlled fashion based on environmental conditions.

For a clinician, this means thinking beyond each step of the methods used to enhance the health of patients and making decisions that achieve beneficial results in the end while consuming the minimum amount of energy along the way (and leaving the transition substrates unharmed). Such thinking is often called outcome analysis when applied to a disease state or to aggregates of patients.

For a chief information officer, it means understanding the strategic goals of the organization on the basis of enterprise structure, subculture make-up, and the environment in which it functions.

For a chief executive officer or a manager, it means understanding critical information-intensive organization processes from start to finish and synchronizing the communities involved in delivering and accepting necessary technology.

Regardless of role, understanding these processes mandates extensive input from user communities affected from the very beginning of the effort, because change begins with design. Influential managers, supervisors, and front-line workers should be involved in the evaluation of current procedures and in the analysis of where and how workflow can be improved with information systems. Involvement of middle managers is crucial, because not only are they often most influential in working with departmental supervisors and employees, but they may also be most susceptible to infobia issues, with potential for inordinately high resistance to change.[6] Users can also be very effective in helping you focus on what you wish specifically to leave unchanged in the process.

Business pathway components require analysis from end to end.

The investment of those who will be affected in the design or the selection of the new system, and the resulting sense of responsibility and ownership, allows trusted coworkers who participated in the design to help with user transition. In this way, intracultural teaching, which facilitates change and assuages fears, can be done by those who are most familiar to the people who will be directly affected.

The more users involved in the creation of the new system, the more likely it is the system will actually be "good" and the greater the chances the "good" system will be accepted.[7,8] The information technology subculture, organization management engineers, and system analysts are all important, of course, but only users can give an adequate feel for the impacts of the technology on operations. A large part of this is encapsulated in the concepts of "usefulness" and "usability," which ultimately equate to user satisfaction.[2] This is really just a matter of common sense, which is why it is so often overlooked. If the user task is to cut wood precisely and the current implement for doing so is a chisel, it makes little sense to design and deliver a hammer rather than a saw, even though the hammer and the chisel do work better together.

Users will help define optimal *ergonomics* and will engender a design that is most likely to satisfy what I call the *Conservation of User Energy Principle (COUEP)*. COUEP states that any changes a user must make to utilize new technology will require energy (and probably time). The initial energy expended must be recaptured in a relatively immediate fashion from the technology if the user is to have any likelihood of continuing with the process. If there is not an overall time/comfort savings resulting from the new technology, change will not occur or will not persist. (If this doesn't make sense to you, reread the portion of this chapter on energy of activation and the bio-transition framework.)

Users involved in design will also help to avoid a mistake that technicians sometimes make by invoking the obnoxiously popular *Pareto Principle* where it shouldn't be applied. The Pareto Principle states, "Significant items in a given group normally constitute a relatively small portion of the total items in the group. A majority of the items in the total will, even in the aggregate, be of relatively minor importance."[9] Also known as the 80/20 law, it can be paraphrased by saying that for 80 percent of the users, 20 percent of the functions will supply complete satisfaction; 80 percent of the development work will be done to satisfy the other 20 percent of the users.

The more users involved in the creation of the new system, the more likely it is the system will actually be "good" and the greater the chances the "good" system will be accepted.

Another twisted application of the principle is that all users will be 80 percent satisfied with the application because they will only find it inadequate 20 percent of the time. This might lead one to cut a few corners, because, after all, if 80 percent of the users are satisfied all the time or all of the users are satisfied 80 percent of the time, that is pretty good.

The *Pareto Paradox* observes: There will be a small group of users who require the undelivered or unsatisfactory subset of functions to perform their job 100 percent of the time. This group will consist of articulate, influential thought leaders who used to feel that the new system was the right thing to do.

The fact that an isolated single activity might take longer than before must be countered with benefits that accrue for operations as a whole. Each step must be viewed in light of the stability provided by the entire process.

If COUEP is met through good design (and education, training, and well-executed support), change to a new system can be accomplished. The resulting elimination of waste, increased efficiency, and capture of energy can provide both the substrate and the resources for the changes to come next. Ongoing attention needs to be kept on the benefits of the system to the entire structure. The fact that an isolated single activity might take longer than before must be countered with benefits that accrue for operations as a whole. Each step must be viewed in light of the stability provided by the entire process.

After analyzing the pathways, the right catalysts for each step in the transformation chain can be selected on the basis of the appropriateness of their binding site for the reactants, their shape and flexibility, their capacity to bring substrates into position, their ability to understand directions, and their sensitivity to feedback from environmental conditions. Please ignore the hard edge on the descriptions of characteristics for the change agents, as they are intended to help you make the biological connection for metaphor purposes. People are not enzymes, and their unique behavioral and interactive human capabilities should be valued above all else; their effects on the change process can be as a room full of enzymes if they are allowed to ply their abilities appropriately.

Construct 2: Manage Activation Energy along the Pathways

Any and all methods possible to provide motivation for change and to decrease the transition energy at each step of the pathway to end product should be exercised. The easiest change process occurs when there is a highly favorable set of conditions for both the pathway participants (reactants) and the facilitators (enzymes)—an environment of trust, shared values, and confident direction and a return of tangible benefits to the organization from the change efforts. This requires constant reassurance, appropriate education, and sufficient user training and support.

Each step taken down a pathway in the interest of the stability of the entire organization also needs to take individual human stability into account, and this must be communicated constantly in words and deeds. If rewards or evaluations, for example, were previously based on individual productivity, they should be shifted during the transition process to favor system adoption and supporting the new environment. (Otherwise, end products are likely to hop the transition hill backwards to the more comfortable and more valued initial state.)

In addition to focusing on those directly involved with the new system, attention should be directed to other groups that might not be immediately involved in using the technology but that will nevertheless be affected by it. Customers (clients, if you prefer) are often in this category. Resistance on their part can be far more potent than internal barriers. Patients, by the way, like the use of computers in most cases.[8]

After analyzing the pathways, the right catalysts for each step in the transformation chain can be selected on the basis of the appropriateness of their binding site for the reactants, their shape and flexibility, their capacity to bring substrates into position, their ability to understand directions, and their sensitivity to feedback from environmental conditions.

Executive leadership must communicate organization goals evangelistically; those same leaders must model willingness to change and back up their commitment with strong support for each of the catalysts who make the process happen. A huge part of the change process is conveying the pain or the gain that mandates change in the first place. Methods of communicating the need for transition range from Draconian "doom and gloom shock therapy" to more incremental methods.[6] The most effective way to impart the necessary impetus is every way possible. (In extreme cases one may require use of *change management consultants*.)

Communication that reduces insecurity, diminishes confusion, or clarifies reasons for taking the trip can mitigate resistance and should be shamelessly overdone. This does not mean asking permission or even building consensus, but it does mean listening, addressing worries, responding to valid objections, alleviating fears, and firmly expressing management cohesiveness and commitment to the process. Executives should emphatically relate the need for change to those colleagues for whom they have the most compatible "active site" and then rely on them to transmit the message to reactants with whom they are most suitably matched. Managers in all domains also need to be visible and supportive to front-line workers; they must express the need for change with passion, commitment, and authority and give the uniform impression that doing business the old way is not an option.

Just as different enzymes are necessary for catalyzing change, so are different approaches needed for community education. In other words, each segment that needs to be kept informed may require different means of communication to ensure understanding. Print media, faxes, e-mail, voice mail, meetings, and one-on-one relations, with consistent emphasis on two-way communication, can all be effective. A newsletter or town-hall meeting might be part of an educational arsenal, but they may not be effective instruments for reaching front-line workers who feel much more comfortable hearing from direct supervisors or others within their group.[6]

Skilled communication in endeavors such as these is particularly important, because complex information systems almost never arrive on schedule; the best approach is to reveal general timelines for deliveries or roll-out and to withhold exact dates until there is a precise basis for deployment.

Skilled communication in endeavors such as these is particularly important, because complex information systems almost never arrive on schedule; the best approach is to reveal general timelines for deliveries or roll-out and to withhold exact dates until there is a precise basis for deployment. Furthermore, users should be helped to understand that computer systems and networks often sputter at startup, that implementation can be rocky, and that delays are inevitable. Honesty is the best policy about these possibilities. Plans for dealing with downtime or disasters during roll-out should be well communicated before beginning. It is not a crime to respond to the question, "When will this be here?" with, "We will deliver no system before its time." (This may not be the correct answer for the steering committee, however.)

Videotapes, video conferences, large impersonal meetings, and long memoranda do little to motivate users or convince communities of the importance of the change. (Imagine the effectiveness of a videotaped lecture on the proper killing and eating of watermelon broadcast to the Worship Center in the Land of the Fools.) Regardless of the method of communication, all parties generally respond well to being allowed to make suggestions and voice concerns; if one asks, however, one should be ready to respond. If there is no realistic intent to respond (and that doesn't mean agree), don't ask; if one decides not to ask, consideration should be given to ditching the entire effort. The simple process of discussing change and soliciting input not only reduces anxiety, but also makes the process real for individuals, and it makes them feel more important.

Training involves education but is distinct from it in many ways. Training aims at skills for use of the new technology and can be started long before actual implementation. Because computer savvy and skills can be acquired through activities that are more fun than work, entertainment-oriented learning software can have the effect of painlessly imparting basics.

Executive leadership must communicate organization goals evangelistically; those same leaders must model willingness to change and back up their commitment with strong support for each of the catalysts who make the process happen.

A somewhat mundane example of this might be the deployment of electronic mail to noncomputer literate users, giving them a new medium for complaining about technology. The electronic messages circulating mean that keyboards and distribution lists are being used, and, even though resistance appears to have increased, real activation energy has been diminished. Of course, one would hope that Flight Simulator™ is not replacing work-related activities completely, but the process of increasing pleasure in association with change is quite valuable.

In preparation for training, it's critical to do a skill-base assessment of the users to be affected. This can accomplished with detailed survey, if the stage for change has been properly set (meaning the imperative for change has been communicated). Classes or other forms of teaching can then be tailored to potential users, whose abilities are likely to assume a normal distribution curve.

Experts may only need brief tutorials or may benefit from *computer-based training*. (I put computer-based training in the general category of videotapes as far as real teaching goes, and it may be downright repulsive to brand-new users.) Others will need small team-based classes or even remedial concentration to successfully get on board. In each group, regardless of ability, training must be aimed as much at mitigating infobia as at the direct use of the hardware and application.

Training for large, complex applications can be the most expensive part of implementation. Not only is there the emotional challenge of overcoming infobia, with its financial impacts from absenteeism, equipment loss or damage, and extended coffee breaks, but there also are direct costs in removing individuals from the workplace for training and replacing them during their classes. This is all in addition to the expense of trainers, training facilities, training manuals, and other documentation. And then there is the dreaded *learning curve*.

The learning curve refers to the fact that, after training, the facility of the users with the system in a production environment is less than perfect, and therefore productivity, by old measures, is diminished for some period.[11] The magnitude of the learning curve will depend on the amount of change in operations that the new system requires, the skill with which education and training have been carried out, and the actual performance of the system that has been delivered.

In brief, the better the infobia management through education, communication, and training, the lesser the consequences of the learning curve on operations and the bottom line. Support of users during this critical early time, in the form of hand-holding trainers, support personnel, and troubleshooters, all of whom must function to minimize the appearance of user incompetence, to instill confidence in the system and its appropriate use, and to nurse the shift from training to maintenance, is essential.

The simple process of discussing change and soliciting input not only reduces anxiety, but also makes the process real for individuals, and it makes them feel more important.

It is important to plan for supporting operations with additional personnel, work shifting, work load reduction, and constant back-patting during what can be a significant reduction in work performance. Failure to support operations during this learning curve can result in sabotage, mutiny, Luddism, and severe disruption of homeostasis.

It is this dedication to supporting change, expending energy to get users over the transition hill, and gradually managing infobia that will allow development of an important support structure within operations. To as great a degree as possible, one wishes to rely on subcultural family to help with system problems (which are often user error), rather than the less favorable *help desk or user services*.

One rather disconcerting factor to be pointed out with respect to supporting operations during the learning curve is that, even though users may be significantly less efficient, they are still using up their physical work spaces 100 percent, so adding people to directly help may not be an option.

An additional critical area in training and learning curve support has to do with integrating technology use with customer interactions. In medicine, for example, the health care provider may not naturally be able to interact with the patient and the computer simultaneously, and an application that requires this may be fatally flawed. Different individual practitioners already have different interaction and listening skills (bedside manner), and if they are less than adept at these techniques, which truly constitute the art of medicine, the computer in the room is not likely to help the patient interaction. Therefore, focus on use of the technology in the presence of the patient (or customer) should be accomplished, ideally with mock situations that allow users to overcome infobia before interacting with clients.

The learning curve refers to the fact that, after training, the facility of the users with the system in a production environment is less than perfect, and therefore productivity, by old measures, is diminished for some period.

Construct 3: Harvest Energy and Realize Gains

Management discipline must be exercised to capture liberated energy from the new pathways in tangible, demonstrable, useful ways for the enterprise. This includes measurable performance improvements, quality or service enhancements, and cost reductions or avoidance. In other words, the new systems and information should measurably improve organization stability and ready it for future environmental challenges. A realistic assessment of the resources required to get over the transition hills and the exact ways in which gains will be harvested from the process must be determined; otherwise, resource expenditures will result in little more than heat. This necessitates cost-benefit and cost-efficiency evaluations and consideration of the energy fluxes at each step of the implementation process.

Not every step in the process has to be energy favorable, sometimes no energy will be harvested from a step, or resources will need to be pumped into a step simply to prepare a reactant for the next cascade; subsequent pathway steps, if well-thought-through, will restore energy balance or yield a net gain for use at a future time. This requires thinking about non-linear networks of causation in addition to more apparent direct chains, which, unfortunately, is most difficult to do under pressure.[12] Energy-expensive steps, if viewed in isolation, may not be particularly attractive, and they are really problematic if one fails to reach the remainder of a proposed pathway. Often, such costly steps are referred to as *enablers*; information technology frequently fits into this category.

It should be borne in mind that death during the transition process due to homeostasis chaos is a discomforting possibility. This is more likely to occur if the energy that accrues to the new information system is not recovered in a way that concretely benefits the business; energy should be used to replenish supplies used during the change process, shunted to other pathways to ensure stability, or stored for dealing with future stresses. This challenge is enormous for managers, and, more often than not, a new information system improves efficiency and operations and achieves its preconceived goals, but the energy seems to vanish, like heat, into the environment. Disciplined energy-recovery tools, or "energy carriers," must be developed simultaneously with new system design and implementation; captured energy must be real, measurable, and demonstrable. The duty of management in this regard is to precisely define where energy will be produced, how it will be captured and accounted for, and where it might be subsequently used. Then, from executive directors through front-line metabolizers, expectations must be laid for guaranteeing energy recovery.

This challenge is enormous for managers, and, more often than not, a new information system improves efficiency and operations and achieves its preconceived goals, but the energy seems to vanish, like heat, into the environment.

One of the most difficult concepts for traditional corporations to convey as they shift to a more integrated and less hierarchical model is the notion that recovered resources are not necessarily the property of the metabolic pathway that generated them. Rather, they are riches that accrue to the organism; subculture success must be rewarded, but integration requires great depth of understanding by all participants of the need to donate harvested resources for use by other elements of the enterprise.

Successful elimination of wasteful efforts or expenditures by implementation of information systems (or other reengineering) often allows a form of energy recovery through the process of *disintermediation*, which means someone who was doing something important before is now doing something redundant or useless and may no longer be necessary. Fear of being "disintermediated" is a huge element of infobia.

Clearly, managers need to be skilled in dealing constructively with such personnel issues and in revealing this message. An announcement that a new system will mean a savings of 100 FTEs and increased company profit is not going to do much to lower activation energy; on the other hand, missed opportunities to harvest gains create disease and can require "amputations." Incentives, job improvements, skill augmentation, retraining, and capitalizing on natural personnel attrition are all preferable ways to reframe energy capture and organization benefits.

Exemplary Management Discipline

In a real-life example of the potential for disciplined energy capture, a new medical imaging information system is purchased to streamline operations in a radiology department. The goal is to reduce paper-related inefficiency, diminish unnecessary duplication of x-rays, collect and monitor workflow and resource utilization data, decrease phone traffic, and improve results communication to patients and clinicians. The value and desirability of these improvements should be generated within or coaxed from the department, which takes a little time.

Managers, supervisors, and organization management engineers should be able to forecast total reduction in expected operating costs and improvement in processes as a result of acquisition of the new system.

Managers, supervisors, and organization management engineers should be able to forecast total reduction in expected operating costs and improvement in processes as a result of acquisition of the new system, if department users participate in the analysis, embrace the possibility of benefits, accept responsibility for successful implementation of the system, and actually budget the savings. If the change process is handled well, the department will be (nervously) willing to guarantee the recovery of energy.

Once this commitment is made, costs will be recovered, and they might not all be attributable to the new system! This energy capture discipline spawns an underappreciated parallel byproduct: new methods of efficiency from rethinking processes that manifest themselves more globally. This parallel thought process pathway is the beginning of a very powerful *positive feedback loop*.

Contrast this scenario with the unenlightened process in which a manager from administration culture decides that medical imaging needs to be more efficient and productive, circumvents the cultural steps necessary to impart the need for the change, ignores infobia, and purchases a flashy system he or she saw at a trade show. The transition energy apex at implementation will surpass timberline, and, even if the summit is actually traversed, no guarantees of energy capture have been exacted from unwilling participants, so actual benefits from the trauma are likely to be minimal. Furthermore, the process of parallel efficiency thinking and stimulation of the positive feedback loop will be supplanted by feelings of loathing for management. Pitchforks will be requisitioned en mass.

A realistic assessment of the resources required to get over the transition hills and the exact ways in which gains will be harvested from the process must be determined; otherwise, resource expenditures will result in little more than heat.

This is the case all too often with turnkey systems; the software performs the functions that someone thinks are necessary, but user participation is ignored, infobia is disregarded, and technocentric methods of implementation and training are employed. (When humans are ignored, the CIO should consider updating his or her résumé.)

Putting It Together

In summary, the ideal change situation is one in which both users and managers perceive a need for information improvement that can be actualized with the expertise and technological know-how of an integrated information technology department. Who initially perceives the need for the system is immaterial, as long as the cultural elements of system evaluation, design, selection, and guarantee of energy savings are sensitively managed.

...the ideal change situation is one in which both users and managers perceive a need for information improvement that can be actualized with the expertise and technological know-how of an integrated information technology department.

Emphasis on pain or pleasure drivers for the change will set the stage for the end state, and, as the joint evaluation and selection process is engaged, communication, education, and forging of solidarity of purpose begins to move the entire community of affected users toward the goal. Infobia issues are met head on by those with the best means of interacting with affected groups or individuals, incentives and evaluations criteria are realigned to support new methods, and commitments for definitive energy harvesting are obtained.

Then implementation proper can begin. Arrangements for training based on initial user skill sets are crafted, support for operations during training and learning curve phases is acquired, and on-site technical support is arranged. Emphasis is placed on minimizing feelings of incompetence, and management gratitude is expressed in a meaningful way. All managers focus on decreasing the energy of transition with each individual, on maintaining the motivation for change, and on selecting appropriate catalysts to enhance the speed of the process. As transition occurs, COUEP kicks in, global rather than provincial perspectives are developed, performance improves, and success is imminent.

The new sense of mastery by users invigorates morale and gives rise to parallel efficiency thinking and activity, and a positive feed-back loop is instigated in which the combination of beneficial end product and harvested energy provides more momentum for ongoing change.

This makes for a very nice synopsis, but there are two items experienced managers are sure of as regards information systems. The first is that, despite all cognizance, planning, empathy, and transition energy manipulation, unexpected results will occur. Technical and human complexities of the process are fraught with risk, and the management art of sensing conditions, applying pressure, rewarding effort, and "flexing" structure in real time is critical to reaching the next level. The second is that the instant everyone is over the hill and cruising down to the desired end state, the discovery is made that the end state is little more than the base of the next transition hill to be climbed.

Anything Else?

I hope that the concepts and terms presented here have conferred some level of linguistic prowess in the area of information systems, an understanding of their potential for business enhancements, and an appreciation of the human factors that influence their acceptance. This knowledge base should reduce infobia to an all-time low and elevate confidence dramatically.

If religiously followed, and a miracle happens, the recommendations and principles set forth here will ensure success in implementing a new, complex information system, which is no small feat for anyone involved. With success, optimism will grow for the inevitable next venture, and, as benefits of transformation are harvested, the evolution will yield possibilities of domination in a niche.

If, however, one makes one tiny omission from the important revelations presented here, failure may occur. As has been pointed out by an expert in failure (which might be an expertise somewhat embarassing to lay claim to), we fail because we tend to make a small mistake here, a small mistake there, and these mistakes add up. Sometimes, we fail to make goals specific enough; other times we plan too elaborately.[12] Even if failure occurs, it will be accompanied by increased insight, knowledge, and aplomb; you will be in excellent company. In the event that you do not experience success the first time around, you should pick up the October 18, 1982, *Time* magazine that is still on the side table at your therapist's office and read author John Updike's assessment.

> *I think what's most disturbing about success is that it's very hazardous to your health, as well as to your daily routine. Not only are there intrusions on your time, but there is a kind of corrosion of your own humility and sense of necessary workmanship. You get the idea that anything you do is in some way marvelous.*—John Updike, American author, 1982.

Success may just be an in term to teach us the value of humility!

References

1. Bridges, W. *Managing Transitions: Making the Most of Change.* Reading, Mass.: Addison-Wesley Publishing Co., 1991.
2. Lorenzi, N., and others. "Antecedents of the People and Organizational Aspects of Medical Informatics: Review of the Literature." *JAMIA* 4(2):79-93, March-April 1997.

3. Watzlawick, P., and others. *Change: Principles of Problem Formulation and Problem Resolution.* New York, N.Y.: W.W. Norton, 1974.

4. Miller, G. *Energetics, Kinetics, and Life.* Belmont, N.Y.:Calif.; Wadsworth Publishing, 1971.

5. Dörner, D. *The Logic of Failure.* Reading, Mass., Addison-Wesley, 1996, p. 6.

6. Dickout, R., and others. "Designing Change Programs that Won't Cost You Your Job." *McKinsey Quarterly*, No. 4, 1995, pp. 101-16.

7. Swanson, E. "Management of Information Systems: Appreciation and Involvement." *Management Science*, 21:178-88, 1974.

8. Ives, B., and Olson, M. "User Involvement and MIS Success: A Review of Research." *Management Science* 30:586-603, 1984.

9. Willoughby, T. *Business Systems.* Cleveland, Ohio: Association for Systems Management, 1981.

10. Brownbridge, G., and others. "Patient Reactions to Doctors' Use of Computers in General Practice Consultations." *Social Science and Medicine* 20(1):47-52, 1985.

11. Horak, B. "Implementation Time Productivity." *Organizational Issues in Medical Informatics*, Oct. 1-2, 1993.

12. Dörner, D., *op. cit.*, p. 33.

Information System Projects

Part 4

Enlightened and enthused by mastery of information system concepts, and energized to become a learner or to create a "learning organization," one may become embroiled in a computer project of some kind. Whether the vision involves a purchase from a vendor, a cooperative development effort with an information technology partner, or in-house program development with the information systems department, more new terminology will be needed. The generic language in this section is important regardless of the area for which the information system is being developed. If one already has experience with technical project management, and if it was typical, it probably did not involve rest, relaxation, and a sense of control. Whether you failed or succeeded, managed the effort or toiled in the trenches, loved or hated the experience, you may still find some subtleties here to enhance your composure during what will be a relentless succession of similar efforts far into the future.

Enormous amounts of money and effort are usually spent on system design and development; methods of maximizing gains from creative work are examined first. Great pressure is subsequently associated

> *Effort is only effort when it begins to hurt.*—José Ortega y Gasset, Spanish essayist, philosopher, 1949.

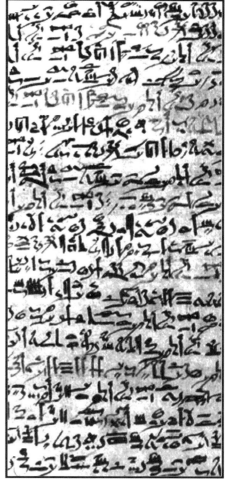

with information system implementation and support, because the costs of the latter dwarf those of development and because individuals building the system are usually enthusiastic about it, in contradistinction to those to whom it is being delivered. (Fundamental concepts of major importance for implementation were reviewed in Part III of this book, and a reconsideration of the psychological, cultural, and transition issues discussed there may be warranted prior to digging into the more concrete processes detailed here.)

Chapter 9

Information System Projects: Planning and Development

Theoretical knowledge is not the same as hands-on knowledge.—Dietrich, Dörner, German author (discussing the Chernobyl incident), 1989.

Prior to describing the information system project life cycle, a general set of pertinent principles:

- First, goals of the effort should be clear and well communicated before beginning.

- Second, adequate time and effort should be spent to understand processes as they exist, and to conceive how they will operate when the goals are achieved.

- Third, project team members should be authorized and prepared to make decisions and to take actions with as few organizational impediments as possible.

- Fourth, constant review and assessment of results along the way should occur, and willingness should be developed to alter approaches or methods when things aren't working.

- Finally, potential system users should be involved in design and development to avoid creating a system for "someone else." This ensures that creators are not shielded from the effects of their creativity, aligning with the wisdom of Herbert Spencer, who observed: "The ultimate result of shielding men from the effects of folly is to fill the world with fools."[1]

Conception and Analysis

The process begins when you or someone you trust gets a bright idea for improving business with better information and formulates a *project vision*. This vision describes the *goals* and reasons for embarking on the work. It will be revisited repeatedly during design and implementation to provide solace for enduring the excruciating tribulations of system development. This vision is evaluated at a *high level* by other managers and enterprise experts in the copy room or at staff meetings, depending on organization culture.

This group is often called a task force, which is ironic, because it usually accomplishes few tasks and generates little or no force.

Consultation of the *enterprise model* that has been developed may occur, or agreement to proceed out of relative ignorance may be subsequently made based on the merits of the idea at a *low level*. High level means general, vague, poorly defined, and not well understood. Low level means very detailed, specific, and clearly defined (but still probably poorly understood).

The manner in which the process occurs depends to some extent on *management style* and enterprise politics, but the probable beginning will be identification of a *project sponsor*, the key visionary responsible for genesis of a project. (Generally, one will saddle the person who came up with the idea with this responsibility, unless, of course, it was your idea.) The project sponsor will gather a group of capable individuals who will do some critical *strategic planning*. This group is often called a task force, which is ironic, because it usually accomplishes few tasks and generates little or no force. Nonetheless, the right people need to perform a *cost-benefit* and/or *cost-effectiveness study* to decide if the idea really has potential as a *project*.

Cost-Benefit versus Cost-Efficiency

Cost-benefit studies are among the most troubling and difficult concepts in management, especially in the realm of information systems; they analyze the cost of acquisition of a system and its predicted economic benefits.[2,3] This quantitative assessment is also referred to as a "return on investment" analysis.

The cost-benefit analysis pales in significance when compared to its gifted sibling, cost-effectiveness analysis. The latter is an evaluation of the cost of acquisition of a system versus the effects on the organization in total, which is much more qualitative, and therefore real, but often immeasurable. It is analogous to assessing a complete metabolic pathway as opposed to a limited series of transition steps or isolated cycles, and it is correspondingly more difficult to quantify.

Much of what information systems users want cannot be proved cost-beneficial but is intuitively cost-effective. For many businesses, these systems are simply "face value" requirements—underpinnings for future quantifiable performance gains that cannot be attained without them. The process of converting qualitative items (i.e., better communication, improved access to information, better decision making, higher quality, fewer wasteful activities) into value equivalents requires expert opinion, usually by *management engineers* or, for the less fortunate, by *consultants*. After time/motion studies, flow structure diagrams, on-site observation, and extensive interviews, usually at great expense, consultants and engineers can turn the ethereal organizational effectiveness benefits into favorable numbers, just long enough to persuade *steering committees* of the strategic advantage of a system.[3]

Buy or Build

If the cost-benefit determination suggests a favorable return on investment, or if the evaluation discovers that the project will establish an *infrastructure* that will be a strategic enabler for the future, the task force may begin the difficult process of deciding whether to buy a *turnkey* system, have the information technology department write the code and put the network together, or enter into a joint agreement with a *partner* to work toward the end goals.

Turnkey systems are supposedly ready to be dropped into an organization and turned on, containing all necessary hardware, software, documentation, and training materials. (Turnkey-lite systems, which include only software and training materials, are referred to as "shrink-wrapped" products.) The expectation with most turnkey systems is that the business processes will adjust to the software. Experience suggests otherwise.

> *The process of converting qualitative items (i.e., better communication, improved access to information, better decision making, higher quality, fewer wasteful activities) into value equivalents requires expert opinion, usually by management engineers or, for the less fortunate, by consultants.*

This process will involve *request for information/request for proposal (RFI/RFP)* and site visits to determine the approach of choice. The RFI is a formal document distributed to a set of vendors as an instrument to gather information about marketplace offerings. It is an early investigative tool that seduces vendors into thinking they might actually be able to compete for an organization's business. The RFP is a similar document generated after the RFIs have been evaluated, setting forth the precise requirements and questions relating to a desired system or service. RFPs are sent to a subset of vendors who are given an opportunity to further specify their offerings, answer the questions, and indicate a bid price for their product. The details of RFPs are strictly confidential to avoid troublesome bickering among contestants.

Each time new information is obtained from these efforts, the cost-benefit studies are revisited to be sure fundamental assumptions and project vision are intact. Based on the RFP results, a decision will be made to buy a package, partner with a vendor for custom development, or embark on the work exclusively within the organization.

If a decision is made to proceed, the task force will give way to a steering committee, which is an interested group of powerful organizational icons whose purpose is to support and guide the efforts of individuals mired in the actual design, development, implementation, and management of the project.

If a decision is made to proceed, the task force will give way to a *steering committee*, which is an interested group of powerful organizational icons whose purpose is to support and guide the efforts of individuals mired in the actual design, development, implementation, and management of the project. If a steering committee is formed, the consultant larvae have an excellent chance of attaining full-fledged commensalism (more on the role of consultants later).

Project Launch

For purposes of illustration, I will pursue a *cooperative development* effort between a company and a vendor-expert-partner, because this process contains the most complexity and reveals unique terminology. It does not imply any difference in the chances of success. Assuming one has selected the partner in the RFI/RFP/site visit process, the project sponsor and steering committee create the project team, led by a *project manager*. Project managers are persons responsible for controlling project scope and for guiding efforts in attaining the *goals* and directives set forth in the *project vision*.

Generally, a single manager is not enough, and one from each partner team will be appointed for balance and equity. Depending on politics in the participating companies, even more than one project manager per side may be chosen to add specific expertise. Regardless of the number of project managers, if there is more than one, a *project executive* from each side will need to be selected.

Project executives are managers who have ascended the ranks of project managers by virtue of dedication, brilliance, wisdom, and indomitable spirit. Individuals in this position are experienced and specially certified in conflict management; they will lose their jobs if the project is not successful. (How this differentiates them from the remainder of individuals on the project who will also lose their jobs if the project is unsuccessful is a great mystery in upper level management.)

Scope and SOW

Now arduous information gathering and negotiating begins to define *functional requirements*, determine the *scope* of effort, and chisel out the all important *statement of work (SOW)*.

The scope is the set of rigidly delimited and carefully described functional contents the parties agree to accomplish in the project.

Functional requirements include descriptions of the precise inputs to the system; processes to be performed by the application; interactions of users with the computer and outputs of the program; and detailed information about the volumes of data to be handled, performance criteria, anticipated network traffic, hardware configurations, and user constraints on the system. Technical elements of the functional requirements may be delineated in a separate technical requirements effort. The process of revisiting, re-evaluating, and reconfirming assumptions made in development of the SOW is sometimes referred to as *due diligence*.

The scope is the set of rigidly delimited and carefully described functional contents the parties agree to accomplish in the project. The costs are estimated for realizing the functional requirements, including hardware, software, networking, testing, and support. After haggling that drags on for months, the statement of work is signed and the project is finally conceived. (One is free to draw biological conclusions about the statement of work process, seeing as how it leads to conception.)

The beginning of a formal project mandates the development of a project plan, which should elucidate critical pathways, define critical success factors and critical enablers, and identify bottlenecks.

Usually, the statement of work mandates a more detailed gathering and refining of requirements, often accomplished through a series of *joint application design (JAD)* sessions, which are hyper-intense meetings of users and development experts. JADs should allow early user involvement in design; this involvement should not be underestimated. Experienced managers may wish to do JAD sessions before the statement of work is finalized, but the risk in this case is that nothing will ever get done.

The Plan

Milestones are used initially in a project to indicate markers of progress, often tied to major deliverables and associated with major payments.

The beginning of a formal project mandates the development of a project plan, which should elucidate *critical pathways*, define *critical success factors* and *critical enablers*, and identify *bottlenecks*.

Critical pathways are series of events in the development that must be completed in order to allow any further progress, and bottleneck describes any of a multitude of points or individuals in a process that limit the rate at which all efforts can proceed. Sometimes, bottlenecks are due to individuals with singular expertise on a project who cannot possibly work any harder or longer without "decompensating." A unique situation involving group bottlenecks, summarized in *Duh's' Principle*, observes that a point of saturation will be reached on the project at which the addition of any new individuals will have an overall damaging effect on progress because of the time it will take to "bring them up to speed." A difficult principle to grasp, it assumes that all current project members are qualified, energetic individuals with superb work ethics and great attitudes who are fully utilized.

The project plan charts the course from design through implementation using graphical tools such as the *Gantt chart*, an almost indecipherable geometric graph/chart hybrid that *plots* tasks in a project by subject area or individual against time. The resulting overlapping bar indicators are used to determine when resources should be added or subtracted, when critical pathways will be negotiated, and when team members are most likely to be calling the crisis hot line. Tasks that must be completed before others can be started are called "critical dependencies" and are supposed to be more obvious in a display such as this.

During longer projects, periodic *replanning* will be mandated. Replanning is enormously draining, as it entails shuffling resources, recreating timelines, swapping managers, and infusing complexity, as well as cessation of actual project work. It is necessitated when the project falls behind schedule. Count on it.

Another fascinating and useful method of diagramming and estimating the project is called *function point analysis*, which breaks functional areas and features down into branching-related granular actions, sometimes to the level of single data field behavior, thus providing a way to size the complexity and potential expense of development. A large project may contain 5,000-10,000 function points, an enormous one, 50,000 or more.

The project plan divides the project into a set of *deliverables* with *releases* and *milestones*, often grouped into phases. Deliverables are items promised to customers. Most deliverables are detailed in the *statement of work*; examples of deliverables in addition to the software itself might include design documents, user guides, training manuals, and even support personnel. A release is a delivery of a software set to testers or users in an unfinished form with a numeric designation that usually contains a decimal and several digits. Releases are sometimes called "versions." As a rule, a higher or more impressive version number (e.g., 5.235) indicates a less satisfactory development process.

Milestones are used initially in a project to indicate markers of progress, often tied to major *deliverables* and associated with major payments. By midproject, these intervals will be replaced by footpebbles and then by inchgrains. A *phase* is a group of tasks, with steps and activities, that, when performed in concert, result in a major set of deliverables. Phase's identical twin, *stage*, can only be distinguished from its sibling if you are their parents.

Players

The beginning of the project also calls for human and financial resource allocation. In addition to the array of managers mentioned above, other human resources to be added include *developers*, *facilitators*, *system analysts*, testers, and documentors, as well as other project support personnel.

Developers write software code in a language that can be compiled and loaded on a computer; they are charged with the enormous responsibility of converting user needs into *programming language* and computer actions. Facilitators are individuals with the responsibility of guiding meeting discussion, monitoring the agenda, mediating conflict, reframing issues, clarifying observations, and managing egos, while at the same time remaining dispassionate and remote. Facilitators are sometimes not directly involved in project issues so that they can remain unbiased in their approach to the problems; a chief duty is to keep participants from going off on *tangents*.

System analysts are uniquely qualified individuals with the gift of accurately evaluating the details of a computer or business system that must be aligned for adequate functioning of the whole. Chief emphasis of these analysts is on exception definition and planning—the art of detailing all conceivable minutiae that could possibly go wrong. Documentors prepare myriad papers, discussed below, and support personnel manage equipment, leave annoying voice-mail, arrange for conference rooms and meetings, make copies, and drop like canaries in a gas-filled mine.

Financial support is referred to as the project budget, tightly coupled with the project plan, which proves conclusively that time is money. At this juncture, the wise executive recalls Golbus' Law: "No major computer system is ever installed on time, within budget, with the same staff that started it, nor does the project fully do what it's supposed to do."[4] The corollary to *Golbus's Law* is: "Yours is unlikely to be the first."

If the powers of the organization are in a beneficent mood, they may provide *contingency funding*, a small amount of money (usually less than 20 percent of a project's budget) set aside for unanticipated needs during the project life cycle.

Development and Testing

The project team decides on a *development methodology* to be used and will continually assess project *risks* and *progress* as things proceed via things called *project status* reports.

Development methodology is a prescribed series of steps or principles to be followed from embarkation on a project to delivery of product, elucidating the path of *iteration*, development, testing, piloting, and user acceptance.[5,6]

Risks are the omnipresent elements of every decision or action that forebode failure, and progress is an elusive mystical phenomenon in large projects that some experts believe does not really exist.[7] Project status reports, which are supposed to measure progress, are confusing graphical displays of project tasks started versus project tasks expected to have started; or tasks expected to be completed versus those actually completed. One should not be offended to hear software developers refer to the project as a *death march*, which is loosely defined as a project that is more than twice as expansive as can be accomplished with alotted time or resources.[8]

Documentation

The development methodology will determine the cycles of design, code, and test, but, regardless of the methodology, an enormous amount of project documentation will be generated: *design documents*, *system documents*, *baseline documents*, *configuration management documents*, *test scripts*, and *user/training guides* are examples.

Design documents are written records of project requirements and intentions of several types:

- Joint application design document *(JAD)*—notes from sessions with users solidifying a set of essential design elements that serve as a basis for crafting the external and internal design documents.

- External design report (EDR)—formal, detailed, extensive, analytic narrative documenting precise requirements for design and development of a function in the application, generally from the user perspective

- Internal design report (IDR)—detailed document similar to the external design document, but distinguished from the former in that it focuses entirely on elements of the information system's internal functions in technically indecipherable language, generally from the developer perspective.

System documents are descriptions of system technical functions and operation at the time of delivery:

- The configuration management systems document (CMS) addresses exactly what kinds of hardware are needed to run an application—how to load, unload, boot, reboot, take down, backup, and solve problems in a system, and steps for monitoring operations and recovering lost files.

- The baseline document charts every function, feature, computer screen, code path, and data object and displays them in microscopic font for all project team members; it serves as the absolute arbiter of what is in or out of scope.

Roles and Responsibilities

Project manager work sessions will be ongoing in an attempt to manage *scope creep* and *project change requests (PCRs)* and to evaluate *problems* and *issues*.

Scope creep is the insidious process of project expansion that adds complexity and cost to the effort. It is the most common reason for not meeting a milestone or deliverable.

Project change requests (PCRs) are critical elements of any project, providing a formal written and tracked mechanism used for partners (or opponents) to present each other with items they believe they should either obtain for free or provide at exorbitant cost during project development. PCRs may be generated by any project participants and be given to the managers, thereby documenting design

> *Scope creep is the insidious process of project expansion that adds complexity and cost to the effort.*

concerns or delivery problems requiring attention. PCRs *may* generate additional costs, or time delays, but they *always* serve to distract managers from real work. There are nuances to PCRs (investigation versus implementation, *issues* versus *defects*, what was said versus what was written down, etc.)

A problem is anything that hinders or prevents achievement of a stated goal, and an issue is a euphemistic term for incomplete comprehension of an aspect of a project, applied when no one can ascertain if another *JAD* session should be convened or more drastic personnel action should be undertaken to solve a new problem.

Disconnect is the name given to the sudden realization that there is no common understanding whatsoever between customers and developers about an element of an application.

The team individuals will vary over time in responsibility and title, depending on deliverables and cycles. For example, system analysts may become *functional area owners (FAOs)* responsible for a prescribed function or set of functions in a development project whose job it is to detect *disconnects* and to ensure application consistency. The process of ensuring consistency is sometimes referred to as *consolidation*. Disconnect is the name given to the sudden realization that there is no common understanding whatsoever between customers and developers about an element of an application.

At very special times during the work, an event called a *project review* occurs. This is a process of critical review of a project by a set of impartial observers for the ostensible purpose of suggesting changes to improve progress and maximize chances of success. Project reviewers are masters of observation and tact and are skilled in discovering from all involved parties how things are really going. They can arrive at any time, but they will always arrive at a time of project crisis.

Testing, Defects, and Bugs

As code is developed and "dropped," it must undergo complex *system testing*, a process of insanely repetitive software manipulations intended to reveal bugs or defects in the code.

Bugs are little idiosyncrasies in software that disallow smooth application function. They are different from *defects* in that they are not always the result of programming errors, but can represent spontaneous mutations in the code. Defects are failures of software to perform as required by external and internal *design documents*.

Code problems of this nature are discovered by the methodical use of *test scripts*, which are prescribed steps directing manipulation of an application to see if it does what it is supposed to do according to design documents. Test script writers are very important, because they translate detailed user requirements into simple execution protocols that any uneducated tester can negotiate. Defects are graded by severity:

- The system completely crashes because of the defect (severity one).

- The system suffers miserably, struggles in agony, gasps, and causes interfaced systems to crumple without completely hosing, and there is no work-around (severity two).

- The system works in an aberrant fashion, requiring extreme work-around measures to circumvent the defect (severity three).

- The system contains misspellings, screen inconsistencies, data errors, and style gaffes that make users pine for a severity one defect (severity four).

Two fascinating varieties of defects are intermittent defects, which occur only under some mysterious circumstances or only in a specific environment (and are therefore very difficult to replicate and fix), and upstream defects, which completely block testers from discovering other defects that would be apparent if they could finish the test script.

There are several varieties of system testing:

- *Internal system testing*—done privately by developers to see how many bugs and defects they expect to deliver.

- *Integration testing*—done by developers and FAOs who attempt to evaluate the function of the code as it relies on interfaces to other systems.

- *Regression testing*—the sometimes automated but always inadequate retesting of all of the code after a defect is fixed because of the likelihood that the repair generated new defects in the software (defined mathematically by: repair = new defects.)[3] This testing must be repeated when any new code is added to existing software.

- *User acceptance testing (UAT)*—begun after the first three steps are solidly completed, utilizing an unsuspecting group of actual users to see how the code performs under conditions approximating production. This area of testing can be expected to surface more *defects* than the number discovered by the combination of all three previous testing methods.

- *Pilot testing*—evaluation of code by actual users in a production environment. It reveals occasional bugs in the software, but, more crucially, it outlines major design and development overhauls deemed mandatory by the testers for widespread user acceptance.

Most of the testing beyond the internal and integration stages occurs after a *confirm step* in which the functions of the application are demonstrated to the customer in order to convince buyers that the code is grossly in line with expectations and to confirm that design elements have been understood.

By the time testing is being done, and periodically during the development process, creative activities and software code become *intellectual property* and arguing over who gets credit for what can begin. At specific times, versions of the code should be carefully dated, notarized, and locked away to guard against other people working on the same type of project accusing you of stealing their ideas.

Prototype

Sometimes a prototype is used during development to give visual credence to the ideas generated in the JAD sessions. A *prototype* is a set of computer screens meant to demonstrate what a user might see in the end product, conveying the idea that the observed manipulations will ultimately actually cause something to happen. This prototype is "fantasy-ware," without architecture, communications, data, or infrastructure to support it.

The prototype is rarely perfect to start with, so redesign and re-prototyping may be undertaken in a process called *iteration*. Actually, iteration is a more general term referring to the act of doing something repeatedly until it is finally right. *Rapid iterative prototyping* describes a unique type of development methodology that is supposed to run through the design-code-prototype-test cycle quickly, such that user input can be rapidly incorporated into the application, particularly when functional requirements are very complex or difficult to define up front. (There is no other English expression I am aware of that describes the situation represented of three incompatible terms placed together to represent a single concept. In other words, rapid iterative prototyping, in a pure form, is presently unworkable.)

A prototype is a set of computer screens meant to demonstrate what a user might see in the end product, conveying the idea that the observed manipulations will ultimately actually cause something to happen.

Pilot

After thorough testing, code may be introduced into a pilot, which refers to the first introduction of new software into a production atmosphere. Pilot users are afforded the opportunity to use the program to be sure there are no problems and to demonstrate application usefulness in the trenches. Pilot releases are often signified by a variety of Greek letters (α-1, α-2, ß-1, ß-2, etc.) that generally connote the relative maturity and readiness of the code for production, with being nearly ready. These releases occur before all bugs and defects are fixed, and so *workarounds* (unnatural steps in a previously smooth operation that users must take to compensate for vagaries of a new software application) are required.

Pilot users judge the product on its *performance* and *system usability*. Performance refers to how quickly a system will execute its intended functions, and usability is the degree to which a system meets the needs of the user community.

Anything Else?

After the complete testing gauntlet has been run, with bugs and defects repaired, a *functional demonstration* is held. This is the glorious time when users, project sponsors, the project team, steering committees, and executives observe the full application with all its functionality running in a special environment. A marvel to behold, the functional demonstration is reminiscent of a graceful school of colorful angel fish, harmoniously darting in perfect unison with each other in dazzling beauty. The code is then deployed to the dry land production environment.

Change means movement. Movement means friction. Only in the frictionless vacuum of a nonexistent abstract world can movement or change occur without that abrasive friction of conflict.—Saul Alinsky, U.S. radical activist, 1971.

References

1.	*Oxford Dictionary of Quotations*, Third Edition. New York, N.Y.: Oxford University Press, 1979, p. 514.
2.	Van Bemmel, J., and Musen, M. *Handbook of Informatics*. Bohn, Germany: Springer-Verlag, 1997, pp. 495-8.
3.	Kian, L., and others. "Justifying the cost of a Computer-Based Patient Record." *Healthcare Financial Management* 49(7):58-67, July 1995.
4.	Worthley, J., and DiSalvio, P. *Managing Computers in Health Care*, Second Edition. Chicago, Ill.: Health Administration Press, 1989.
5.	Yourdon, E., and Constantine, L. *Structured Design: Fundamentals of a Discipline of Computer Program and Systems Design*. Upper Saddle River, N.J.: Yourdon Press/Prentice-Hall, 1978.

6. Waters, K., and Murphy, G. *Systems Analysis and Computer Applications in Health Information Management*. Germantown, Md.: Aspen Systems Corp., 1983.

7. Horgan, J. "The End of Progress." In *The End of Science*. New York, N.Y.: Broadway Books, 1997, pp. 9-31.

8. Yourdon, E. *Death March: The Complete Software Developers Guide to Surviving Mission Impossible Projects*. Englewood, N.J.: Prentice-Hall, 1997.

Chapter 10

Information System Projects: Implementation and Support

Failure does not strike like a bolt from the blue; it develops gradually according to its own logic. Dietrich Dörner, German author, 1989.

Implementation and support issues outlined here are based on the deployment of a large-scale integrated system, because that was what was designed and developed in chapter 9. (Smaller scale system roll-outs will involve a subset of the elements presented here, but just because things may be "skinnied down" doesn't mean they will be any easier to accomplish.) All parties involved in managing roll-out and support of information systems have every right to be terrified on the inside, but mastery of the vocabulary and the ideology that follow should allow them to appear supremely confident. Remind the CEO or president (if you aren't one) that catalysts of change are not supposed to be destroyed in the process (see Chapter 8). Leave a copy of this book, liberally highlighted, on his or her desk.

The ways in which corporate life is expected to change after implementation (losses, gains, opportunities) should be communicated, along with empathy for the stress and chaos inherent in the change. This is generally referred to as education, but do not use this term publicly, because it reminds people of school, which increases anxiety.

Communication

Early on during selection or development of an information system, *change management procedures* to ensure user ownership of the apocalypse that is about to reign should be undertaken. As delivery time nears, detailed planning should be done to define the communication methods that will keep everyone abreast of events. Messages delivered should be matched to the receptivity of the audience to be influenced. Communication should be consistent and inclusive (customers, community, legislature, unions, etc.), because complex information systems can have far-reaching indirect effects. The ways in which corporate life is expected to change after implementation (losses, gains, opportunities) should be communicated, along with empathy for the stress and chaos inherent in the change. This is generally referred to as *education*, but do not use this term publicly, because it reminds people of school, which increases anxiety.

Commitment of management to implementation should be clear in all communications. When a firm schedule can be established, it should be tactically disseminated. It is better to announce delivery dates to targeted audiences than to making sweeping, organization-wide announcements, unless there is 100 percent assurance of delivery.

Users are unimpressed when they are suddenly unable to do what they used to do because you have upgraded their system.

User concerns should be elicited and discussed directly, with reassurances that the interests of the "changees" are at heart. The most effective communication technique of all is a presentation of the system itself (or of a *prototype*), along with a convincing rendition of the benefits of switching to it, with ample time for user participation, questions, and feedback.

Much of the communication methodology will depend on user readiness to work with the new technology and data and on the resources and emphasis the company is willing to place on training and support during the learning process, particularly with regard to the costs of decreased productivity during transition.

Technical Infrastructure Establishment

Detailed plans for "actualizing" the system architecture should be depicted in the *functional requirements*. Precise *site preparation* provisions need to be defined and facility impacts considered, including workstation, server, network hardware, cabling, and environmental conditions issues. Floor and desk-top space assessments, electrical outlet availability, phone/network connection jack locations, power supply regulators (*uninterrupted power supply, UPS*), heating, ventilation, air conditioning (*HVAC*), lighting, fire protection, and physical site security all need to be accounted for.

Ergonomic factors may drive the physical location of hardware within the work environment as well as within the building; the possibility of equipment damage during use and of breaches of physical security or information privacy and designs for optimization of user comfort and efficiency are all considerations. No matter how well you prepare for this, rollouts in the clinical environment will inevitably result in some computers being installed in sinks. This is not done to make the deployment team look ridiculous, but rather to point out that there really is no other place for the equipment in the examination room. The upside of such gaffes is that, when the application actually runs, the customer can be nothing other than amazed.

Prior to deployment, precise definition of *platform configuration* should be established. This includes hardware configuration (computer models and capabilities), software configuration (operating system, authorized applications, use parameters), peripheral device configurations and drivers (monitors, multimedia, input devices, modems), and network configuration (*topology*, *protocols*, media, operating software).

Predelivery preparation (PDP) includes things such as placing purchase or lease orders and receiving; unpacking; assembling; configuring; testing; and, in some cases, repackaging and moving systems to the work site. Transportation and storage of the equipment, on-site set-up, and asset management are elements of site preparation as well. Asset management includes identifying, labeling, and accounting for each hardware item. It also entails disposing of equipment, tracking software licenses and warrantees, and attending to taxes and insurance.

At this time, consideration should be given to organization policies for handling *upgrades* of components and software, for dealing with unauthorized equipment or software use, and for protecting system set-up alterations by well-meaning, or not so well-meaning, hackers in the user community. In addition to establishing an orderly installation schedule that minimizes operational disruption, consideration should be carefully given to the manner in which information and programs on current systems will be preserved and to how use of the new system may affect them, and vice versa. Users are unimpressed when they are suddenly unable to do what they used to do because you have upgraded their system.

In the case of new, large, complex, or radically different applications, user training is best started with an assessment of baseline individual preparedness.

Timing of component delivery is important, because one can count on the fact that users will either begin to use the equipment before it is ready or will refuse to use it when it is actually ready because "it's been sitting there too long, and I forgot how." It may not always be possible to synchronize just-in-time training to avoid problems such as these. A sure way to gain immediate use of a system is to deliver the hardware and the application but forbid its use. (Trust me, this works, but don't try it until you are sure the system is stable and ready to go.)

User Training

In the case of new, large, complex, or radically different applications, user

---

training is best started with an assessment of baseline individual preparedness. Use of a survey (least expensive) or individual one-on-one interviews (most expensive) can help you determine user preparedness. Surveys are generally most productive and efficient; they should not be completely anonymous, or it will be impossible to target training appropriately.

> *It is unwise to leave training plans solely in the hands of technologists, because operations managers should be involved in proactively readying for replacements and operations support during training and the subsequent learning curve.*

Regardless of the method used, gather information in two areas: initial technical skill sets (comfort levels with specific hardware and software, user interface styles, amount of computer use at home and work, understanding of computer terminology, and other details more precisely determined by the exact application to be delivered) and attitudes toward information systems (ability of computers to benefit work processes; capacity of systems to enhance productivity; efficiency or job satisfaction; importance of computing for organization function and potential for miraculous, improved, worsened, or disastrous effects on day-to-day work; positive or negative past experiences with such systems; and trust in information and its use).

Based on user assessments, design training to optimize both learning and system acceptance. The best methods involve "just enough" training rather than regimented uniform curricula that may overwhelm some, bore others, and permit toxic attitudes to pollute the outlook of more confident, malleable, or well-adjusted trainees. Focused and tailored training speeds transition, accelerates positive feedback loop formation, and enhances the rate at which benefits for the company can be realized.

The training group makeup and size should be designed to make users socially comfortable learning while building relationships around the process that will allow support in the production environment. Doctors, for example, may need to be kept with colleagues initially, but, further down the line, interactions with the team and support staff will become critical.[1] (The rationale for this approach is clarified in Chapter 8.)

Choices range from large classroom settings; to individual tutoring; and, in some cases, to *computer-based training (CBT)*. (I am not a strong believer in CBT as a sole method, if for no other reason than that most users who might benefit can be potential positive change agents in classes of other users with initially flawed attitudes.) Training in appropriate groups can build camaraderie as well as skill, which is unlikely to happen while sitting alone with the training disc.

Depending on the magnitude of cognitive and cultural changes required and users' initial skill sets, training can be diluted or concentrated. Long sessions or classes can be detrimental, because absorption and retention of technical skills tend to decline dramatically after a couple of hours. Additionally, users learn best by doing, rather than by being instructed, so the combination of brief but thorough instruction with immediate application use is optimal. Training without immediate access to doing is of limited utility, which is where the term *just-in-time* training originates.

It is unwise to leave training plans solely in the hands of technologists, because operations managers need to be involved in proactively readying for replacements and operations support during training and the subsequent *learning curve*. Support of new users in the production environment often requires creativity, because there may be no physical way to add help during the learning curve phase when workers are 100 percent present but potentially much less productive.

A training environment in which mistakes can be made, sample data can be accessed, and actions can be undertaken during learning that approaches real-life operations to as great a degree as possible can be a great challenge with highly integrated systems where legacy computers are linked together.

Trainers should be excellent teachers, selected for their communication abilities, their understanding of specific cultural and psychological issues, their flexibility, and their ability to inspire trust while imparting knowledge. Of course, they have to know the application, and they require well-done user training guides that are consistent with the user manuals in the production environment. They should be obviously associated with enthusiastic individuals from the occupational communities and subcultures receiving training. This association provides fearful trainees with a friendly and familiar link to the teacher.

Skill levels, attitude, and company resources will determine whether in-house trainers or contracted teachers are used, where the training will occur (which may drive facility changes), and the degree of expense that will be incurred to create practice environments for initial as well as ongoing training. The time-frame for roll-out, the urgency for switching to the new system, the possibility of running *dual systems*, and the impact of training on different operational departments will help establish the training methodology as well.

Leaders and Training Support

It is very smart to train supervisors, managers, and executives first, so that they can knowledgeably participate in the training of others, even if this only means being present in shifts for short periods at training sessions. Suffice it to say, both senior and mid-level managers must communicate the value of the system and promote transition to it.

A unique and effective alternative method of demonstrating leader support is to have managers and executives fill operations positions while trainees are learning. This accomplishes several goals:

- It demonstrates the dedication of leaders to the difficult change process and displays the regard management has for the success of day-to-day operations.

- It amazes trainees, thereby improving their attitudes toward management initiatives in general.

- It brings executives closer to front-line conditions and customers and generates new insights into potential process improvements from a more believable perspective of direct experience.

- Most important, it makes managers glad that they are managers, and it makes employees glad the managers are managers because of the "clean up" they have to endure when they return from training.

Everyone's attitude generally improves.

Delivering the Application

Take care when serially delivering functions that ultimately work together. If those that require minimal effort and give maximal benefit are delivered before those that are equally necessary but involve more energy to master, the overall risk of failure may rise.

Once the equipment is readied and users are trained, the momentous flipping of the switch occurs. Whether groups of users are expected to use the system following each training session or a delay is necessary, as in the case of a *big bang* approach, depends on the size and the complexity of the application, the degree of integration of the system with other systems, and the amount of zeal managers have for the just-in-time concept. Clearly, if everyone has to go *live* on the system in order for groups or individuals to use the application, the decision about switch flipping will be different from the case where everyone can use the functions in isolation, in which case a gradual addition of users is an option.

The timing decision may also be affected by the requirement of running a *parallel* system during transition (so-called *dual systems*), the potential for sequestration of information on the new system from use by individuals who are not yet on-line, experience with network reliability and system availability, the impact of the learning curve, and the basic structure of the organization.

Sometimes applications are so large or complex that they must be delivered in steps or *releases*. Take care when serially delivering functions that ultimately work together. If those that require minimal effort and give maximal benefit are delivered before those that are equally necessary but involve more energy to master, the overall risk of failure may rise.

Human behavior suggests that the transition may be more troublesome if the end state of the process is relatively less desirable for users because the starting point was prematurely favored by a prior delivery. In stepwise processes, it may be prudent to deliver benefits with efforts simultaneously, such that each transition carries its own reward. This is in contrast to delivering the rewards up front and then expecting selfless dedication to later "pain" without apparent immediate "gain." I call this the *responsibility-reward principle*. The balance between the risk of failure at each transition step and the risk of not completing the entire pathway is important, because the hazards associated with failing to harvest gains from the complete cycle are significant from an organization perspective.

Human behavior suggests that the transition may be more troublesome if the end state of the process is relatively less desirable for users because the starting point was prematurely favored by a prior delivery.

Flexibility in the rate of implementation of large-scale integrated systems is important, because truly accurate predictions about performance are almost never possible and adjustments will be required. Discovery of problems that could never have been anticipated will be made, and it is critical that a support team of on-site technical troubleshooters and "hand holders" be present to support users during application delivery. More important than anything else are fallback procedures for use by operations during the vicissitudes of the transition.

Supporting and Maintaining the System

There are two flavors of user operational support. The first involves direct help with learning, troubleshooting, confidence building, and skills enhancement in the production environment and is called *application support*. The second involves sustenance of the hardware, software, and networks so that the system is available to the users and is called *technical support*. The structure and magnitude of each kind of support may vary, depending on whether a system is in a start-up (roll-out) stage with freshly trained users, new networks, and early version code or in a more stable ongoing steady state. You should immediately question the concept of *steady state*, given what you know about the information age.

Application and User Support

The support of users at roll-out has been touched on already, but attention to *learning curve* issues can't be emphasized enough. On-site hand holding is critical while system competency is gained and the application is stabilized; intracultural operations super-users are the best resources for this purpose, at all shifts if possible, with immediate higher level back-up on call.

It is not acceptable to require that minor issues having to do with user education be handled exclusively through a *help desk*, because timing is critical, interventions are usually simple, and incompetence issues are more sensitively handled by colleagues than by strangers (see the relevant discussion of incompetence issues in Chapter 6).

> *It is not acceptable to require that minor issues having to do with user education be handled exclusively through a help desk, because timing is critical, interventions are usually simple, and incompetence issues are more sensitively handled by colleagues than by strangers.*

The system itself can help in this regard by giving users understandable error messages and directions for getting back on track. Good written user guides and cheat sheets are mandatory, because many users will not wish to reveal their perceived ignorance and would rather solve their problems themselves. The keys here, both in start-up and in steady state, are to help users appreciate the overall system benefits, to minimize frustration, to monitor the emotional state of users, and to inform people of changes in system availability preemptively if scheduled down time is needed or if outages are reported.

In the event of system failure, rapid diagnosis and remedy are critical. Fallback procedures during treatment must be readily available and easily understood by users, and attention should be given to getting information gathered during down times back into the live system. If a failure is hardware-based, there should be "hot spare" replacements immediately available, along with personnel to expediently exchange them (the so-called *hot swap*). This applies to devices at any site, not just computers or workstations at the user junction. At steady state, software applications as well as hardware and networks need to be supported, because bugs and defects will be uncovered and upgrades or modifications will be required.

Application support includes incentives and rewards for system use; sensitivity in recognizing the efforts involved in the change; attention to *ergonomic*, health, and safety issues; and ongoing accommodations for impaired or disabled users. Management engineering can be helpful in evaluating work processes in the new system environment and in responding to user suggestions about better ways to get things done with the new tool. Support of positive feedback thinking is very important.

The *help desk* is the interface between application support and technical support; it is the point of contact for users who are encountering difficulties that cannot be addressed by on-site support users. The help desk must be readily available constantly during system operation, and it must be responsive, helpful, and easily accessible. It should be viewed as a *single point of contact (SPOC)* for users, regardless of the nature of the difficulty the user has encountered.

Rigorous service levels must be determined and adhered to by this important entity, including careful monitoring of the speed with which calls are answered, effectiveness of problem resolution, satisfaction of users with responses, and appropriateness of contacts to the help desk.

Users are new and very important company "customers," and help desk personnel should be able to courteously deal with hardware or software difficulties on all systems, to access higher level resources for problem solving quickly when necessary, and to dispatch technicians to problem sites in a rapid and nonbureaucratic fashion.

Finally, application support involves management courage, in that abuses of the system, security or confidentiality violations, unreasonable recalcitrance, sabotage, or other forms of unhealthy rejection must be dealt with swiftly and firmly.

Other elements of help desk function include collection of data on user and system problems; handling of user requests for moving, adding, or changing things *(MACs)*; and referral of nonsystem-related complaints (which will definitely be received) to a single designated operational resource. Help desk individuals should also be able to interpret and explain system-related enterprise policies and should initiate contacts with users when system changes are to be made or predictable inaccessibility is anticipated.

Finally, application support involves *management courage*, in that abuses of the system, security or confidentiality violations, unreasonable recalcitrance, sabotage, or other forms of unhealthy rejection must be dealt with swiftly and firmly.

Technical Support

Technical support focuses on supporting and repairing the system infrastructure, monitoring system performance, and preventing or predicting technical problems. Within the information systems department, the groups who perform these functions are often called *systems administrators* or computer operations support; they are also responsible for distributing software; configuring hardware; monitoring network parameters; moving, adding, or changing system elements (MACs); backing up critical data; and recovering from problems or disasters. In the distributed client server world of computing, change requests to existing components occur almost constantly, and methods and policies for handling them should be defined from the outset.

Preventive maintenance of the programs and development of procedures for emergency code fixes should be planned. Networks require extensive ongoing attention as well, with security auditing, performance monitoring, availability assessment, and disaster recovery management being key elements. Network capacity should be tracked and managed, performance timed, and the need for reconfigurations or expansions evaluated.

Anything Else?

I believe I've had about enough of this. You?

For the things we have to learn before we can do them, we learn by doing them; men become builders by building and lyre players by playing the lyre.—*Aristotle, Greek Philosopher, 350 BC.*

Reference

1.   Riley, R., and Lorenzi, N. "Gaining Physician Acceptance of Information Technology Systems." *Medical Interface* 8(11):78-90, 82-3, Nov.1995.

Ending with a Win

My theory of evolution is that Darwin was adopted.—Steven Wright, American comedian, 1995.

The following very brief synopsis of the parallel changes that are occurring in health care, information technology, and clinical information systems is designed to emphasize and reinforce the gains you have made in understanding health enterprise subcultures, regardless of your point of origin. It is intentionally laden with the language presented in this book, but in a more concrete and less metaphorical format.

Dr. Iatros' case history gave a more complete view of the philosophical, cultural, and information-based challenges facing the U.S. care delivery process than the distilled points in figure 1, page 198. (The need for universal access to medical information at any point of contact was dwelled upon, as was the need to gather accurate comparable clinical information about disease entities and interventions and to distribute reminders and guidelines to help clinicians deliver rational, more standardized care, based on sound scientific evidence.) These are items that enterprise leaders should anticipate, whether they are directly involved in the health industry or indirectly involved as purchasers of coverage for their employees. (In fact, many practitioners have yet to acknowledge these impending changes.) Technologists and managers need to understand this clinical migration and engage caregivers directly in order to heal the health care system and improve the well-being of the populace.

Clinicians and managers, on the other hand, must understand the enormous challenges that confront information technology experts, a few of which are outlined in figure 2, page 199. If you started this book with little or no basic knowledge of information systems, you should take a moment to congratulate yourself on your ability to comprehend the listed terms and concepts. If you are in administration or a position of executive leadership, you might additionally appreciate what it is you are spending millions of dollars on, and why.

Clinicians, administrators, and technologists must congruently understand what their union truly needs to produce in the way of functional clinical information systems. Some aspects of these systems are summarized in figure 3, page 200. Just as there are many extremely "cool" things that technologists are capable of delivering that have no clinical value, there are more mundane things that they could develop of enormous importance, if only clinicians will help them determine what they are. (Business leaders will spend a great deal of money on the solutions either way.)

Figure 4, page 201, crystallizes the key points of this book by illustrating that winning clinical system development depends on successful migration of inhabitants of the corners of the "health care triangle" toward each other. All of the groups will face significant natural barriers to understanding one another. Some of these barriers will be organizational (bureaucracy, committee structure, human resources policy, structure, politics), some will be cultural (modes of communication, thinking, working, playing, interpreting), and many will be personal (fears, prior experiences, values, biases).

Liaisons assigned to scale the walls and convince one group or another that it must take a particular action are likely to become exhausted and ineffective very quickly. (Go-betweens, unlike catalysts, are often extinguished, if not by the disparate groups then by the vapid results of their efforts.) Nothing short of elimination of the barriers is a requirement for fiscally responsible progress.

The degree to which disparate health organization subcultures can move together to mutual understanding and goal attainment determines the enterprises that will enter the winner's circle. The highest likelihood of success is achieved when clinicians and technologists are intimately involved in strategic and practical enterprise planning and cognizant of what it takes to remain financially solvent, when technologists and business leaders are immersed in the care environment, and when managers and clinicians have developed first-hand reverence for the painstaking process of turning ideas into software. Success also relies on members of each group understanding that expenditures to acquire and support the technology are justifiable only if necessary modifications of practice behavior and decision making are guaranteed and that any technology acquisitions that foster or enable wasteful or useless practices are obviously destructive.

Finally, and of paramount importance, is recognition that patients must participate in both the clinical and the information system challenges. Individuals seeking health must educate themselves about their roles in the excesses and the futility of current practices; participate in prevention processes (when they are well grounded); question recommendations, tests, and treatments in light of this knowledge; and embrace the promise information technology has in their health care future. This patient group adds a third dimension to the "triangle," thus creating a "pyramid of health care," with the fourth corner inhabited by care receivers (figure 5). They obviously will face the same barriers that challenge the other groups as they clamor toward the "sphere" of success.

Anything Else?

Thanks for "listening."

Let us settle about the facts first and fight about the moral tendencies afterwards.—
Samuel Butler, British author, 1880.

Figure 1

Parallel Changes
Health Care

From

- One-on-one provider-patient care
- Illness-focused intervention
- Isolated practitioners and services
- Coding and standards only for billing and claims
- Highly variable practice patterns
- Third-party fiscal responsibility for costs
- Purely economic practice restrictions or guidelines
- Empirical and litigation phobic decision making

To

- Group care visits with prevention/self-care focus
- Population health management and intervention
- Automatically coded, clinically accurate care documentation
- Rapid deployment and acceptance of evidence-based best practices and guidelines
- Fiscal accountability of caregivers and patients for intensity of services, compliance, and shared decision-making

Figure 2

Parallel Changes
In Information Technology

From

- Mainframe applications
- Workstation-based "fat clients"
- Relational database and code language
- Isolated specialty subsystems (lab, pharmacy, imaging, etc.)
- Stand-alone expert/reference/protocol systems
- Relatively primitive security/confidentiality technology

To

- N-tier client server, fault tolerant replicated distributed system architecture
- Integrated seamless subsystem incorporation (interface engine)
- Object-oriented programming
- Industry standard protocols for inter-process communication (HL-7, SGML, TCP/IP, etc.)
- Internet/intranet network access
- Evolved security/cryptography systems for confidentiality and data integrity
- Tool-based (component) functionality
- AI/logic support capability
- Knowledge-based technology tools

Figure 3

Parallel Changes
In Clinical Information Systems

From

- Isolated order/results, practice management, patient demographic, reporting and ancillary services
- Disparate niche proprietary medical record systems
- Monolithic mainframe or PC-based homegrown medical record systems running in parallel with standard paper records.
- Idiosyncratic, hard-coded, inflexible nonstandardized terminolgy
- Unstructured uncoded care documentation via text entry or dictation
- Poor security and confidentiality

To

- Comprehensive complete patient-centered computerized medical records
- Structured codified care documentation
- Real-time-linked electronic order entry and result reporting
- Common Standardized medical terminology for documentation, electronic communication, and synchronous and asynchronous decision support
- Data warehouse (central repository) for analysis and outcomes research
- Flexible, complete user modifiable charting systems with auto matic documentation of activity
- Integrated alerts, reminders, and guidelines for evidence-support ed care.
- Work-flow, task management, and clinical messaging capabilibilies
- Team-oriented software processes to maximize communication and efficiency
- Capability for direct patient/clinical system interaction
- High security and auditability of user access and activity

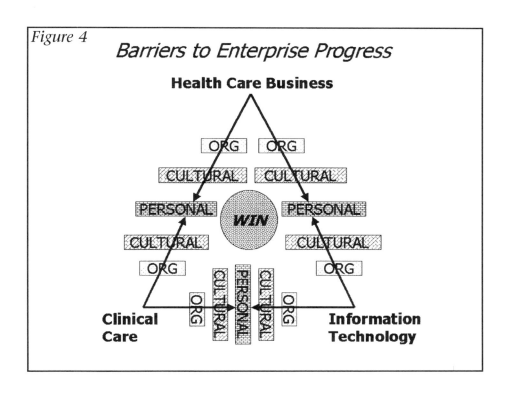

Figure 4

Barriers to Enterprise Progress

Health Care Business

ORG   ORG

CULTURAL   CULTURAL

PERSONAL   *WIN*   PERSONAL

CULTURAL   CULTURAL

ORG   ORG

ORG   CULTURAL   PERSONAL   CULTURAL   ORG

Clinical Care   **Information Technology**

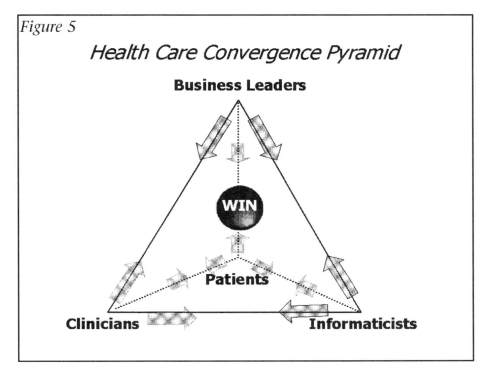

Figure 5

Health Care Convergence Pyramid

Business Leaders

WIN

Patients

Clinicians   **Informaticists**

I have tried in this book to demonstrate that what appear to be contrasting and unrelated subjects may be dealt with productively when juxtaposed and examined together. In fact, the comparison of "inanimate" advanced information system technology and "natural" biological processes makes great sense; both are complex, widely variable in function, diversely integrated, heavily reliant on messages, and subject to tight regulation. Both buck entropy.[1]

It's not unique to medicine that technology has been indiscriminately used with respect to its effect on the environment within which we maintain our "homeostasis." Activist and economist Jeremy Rifkin accurately observed that: "Every technology ever conceived by the genius of human kind is nothing more than a transformer of energy from nature's storehouse. In the process of that transformation, the energy flows through the culture and the human system where it's used for a fleeting moment to sustain life (and the artifacts of life) in a nonequilibrium state. At the other end of the flow, the energy ends up as dissipated waste, unavailable for future use."[2] In other words, our sense of connection with life forms of all kinds and with the energy that supports us in our global medium represents an important extension of the biological enterprise models presented here.

It is absolutely true that a patient is far more than an intricate machine for us to explain and fix; I agree completely with the observation that exclusive and single-minded pursuit of science is detrimental to the relationship between patients and physicians, between scientists and clinicians, and between the medical profession and the public.

Another important and enlightening juxtaposition is that of science and humanity in health care. Using information technology to reshape the "content" of care and clinicians' decision-making processes is necessary to eliminate wasteful activities, but it will not be sufficient for the transition to more appropriate disease management in our age. For America in particular, where the individual and individuality are so highly valued, a shift in thinking, feeling, and acting to a more integrated, community-based view of health (of humans with each other and with the environment) will require a significant cultural change.[3]

I readily admit that the emphasis of this work is unbalanced in the great scheme of healing, but I assert that it is the responsibility of care providers to focus badly needed attention on the evidence for our interventions. It is absolutely true that a patient is far more than an intricate machine for us to explain and fix; I agree completely with the observation that exclusive and single-minded pursuit of science is detrimental to the relationship between patients and physicians, between scientists and clinicians, and between the medical profession and the public.[4] Equally important in the healing process are the role of clinician as humanitarian; the requirement for a deep understanding of the culture and beliefs of the patient, and a similarly deep understanding of our own biases, fears, and attitudes toward practice.[4]

Francis Peabody made the observation in 1927 that "the treatment of disease may be entirely impersonal; the care of a patient must be entirely personal."[5] In this book, I have emphasized tools and methods for improving our approach to disease, because I believe such emphasis elevates the quality of our interventions. The improvements that will accrue to better use of information will not allow relaxation of our responsibility to be compassionate human beings or neglect of the importance of "caring" in healing. Our profession's future depends on the skill with which we compassionately do the right things for our patients, and no longer simply on our bent for doing things right.[6] The right things will not always be what our patients want, or what we were taught, but evidence will supply the courage we need to change our actions and our patients' expectations.

The Sufi teaching story that introduced the principles of understanding culture as a prerequisite for catalyzing change is relevant to almost every aspect of this book, but it is of particular importance to facilitating positive change. There is another Sufi instruction that is specifically applicable to health care today, having to do with three gates through which anything one wishes to say should pass affirmatively before being uttered. The first gate inquires, "Is it true?" The second gate asks, "Is it necessary?" And the final gate queries, "Is it kind?"

The case presentation clearly reveals the importance of discovering what is true in medical practice, using tools and methods of logic and reason. Knowing the truth is a prerequisite to answering affirmatively to the second gate question about the necessity of care interventions. The third gate question, about kindness, is a reminder that medicine is a social and supportive endeavor and that much about healing and health is spiritual and "nonscientific."

Permit me to repeat myself: science is important, but insufficient as an end in itself, because it explains how nature works, but not why.[7-9] The understanding of why is very personal, very powerful, and very important for health care professionals. Although this book has concentrated on elements of importance at the first two gates, it doesn't mean to imply that the third gate isn't a critical one.

A pertinent comment was made late in life by the brilliant author Aldous Huxley, who detailed the inherent nightmarish potential of an ill-managed, hyper-technical existence in *Brave New World* when he observed: "It is a bit embarrassing to have been connected with the human problem all one's life and find at the end that one has no more to offer by way of advice than "Try to be a little kinder."[10]

References

1. Rifkin, J. *Entropy*. New York, N.Y.: Bantam Books, Inc., 1980.
2. *Ibid.*, p. 79.
3. Starr, P. *The Social Transformation of American Medicine*. Basic Books/Harper Collins, 1982.
4. Williams, M., and Roning, C. "Vitruvian Man: Metaphor of a Compleat Physician." *The Pharos*, Summer 1997, pp. 22-7.
5. Peabody, F. "The Care of the Patient." *JAMA* 88(12):877-82, March 19, 1927.
6. Konner, M. *Medicine at the Crossroads*. New York, N.Y.: Vintage Books, 1993.
7. Feynman, R. *QED*. Princeton, N.J..: Princeton University Press, 1985, p. 10.
8. Williams, M., and Roning, C., *op. cit.*, p. 25.
9. Crichton, M. "Postscript: Skeptics at Cal Tech." *Travels*. New York, N.Y.: Ballantine Books, 1988.
10. Fadiman, C. *The Little Brown Book of Anecdotes*. Toronto, Ontario, Canada: Little Brown and Co., 1985, p. 295.

Dictionary, n. A malevolent literary device for cramping the growth of a language and making it hard and inelastic. This dictionary, however, is a most useful work.— Ambrose Bierce, American author, 1958.

This section presents the language of information systems. In it you will find essential terminology for understanding today's technical world of hardware, software, and networks and for communicating with members of project teams who are attempting to use technology to improve organization performance. Also included are biological concepts relevant to this book's discussions of organizational structure and change.

The computer and technology terms often have nuances that are quite entertaining, but even more humorous are the subtleties of language employed by project managers, planners, support personnel, and system developers. (Much of their jargon is also applicable to endeavors outside the realm of information systems.)

The flourishes that accompany the definitions are intended to amuse you, to add a sophisticated sheen to your verbal persona, and to instill a deeper appreciation of the potential risks and benefits of using the words in conversation. They generally resonate profoundly with individuals experienced in the areas of information systems development and project management.

A cautionary note: Communicating the comical undertones of the terms is often useful in relieving tension and improving morale, but there are some unfortunate humorless individuals who just don't "get it." If such individuals work for you, they should be fired. If you work for them, read and enjoy the definitions in private, use them to your quiet advantage, and rejoice in your deeper understanding.

Lexicon[1,2]

A

ABEND: An acronym for Abnormal End of Task, which occurs when a software task encounters an error that is irreparable and that mandates starting over. **Sometimes called codus interruptus.**

Active X: A new technology from Microsoft that, like Java, allows application exchange over the Internet, handling objects and allowing interactive program use between a server and a client accessing it over a network.

activation energy: In biology, the minimal amount of energy needed to bring reactant or substrate molecules into an activated condition (transition state), from which state a reaction will continue spontaneously. The amount of energy needed to get over a "transition" hill that exists between one stable state and another. In business, it is the effort required to achieve change (also called transition). It is really better known as "resistance."

ADP: Adenosine diphosphate, a molecule that functions as an energy carrier in metabolic pathways. It consists of a nucleotide (adenine, which is also one of the four key molecules of DNA), a sugar (ribose), and two of a possible three phosphate groups. It stores energy in its additional phosphate group chemical bond, which it harvests from enzymatic steps in metabolic pathways, in which case it is ATP, or cleaves off the phosphate group to liberate the energy of the bond to donate to a metabolic step and returns to its diphosphate state. It is analogous to the key business concept of management discipline, the ability to harvest true benefits from a business transition for use elsewhere in the enterprise.

ADSL: (see asymetric digital subscribe line)

A.I.: (see artificial intelligence)

algorithm: A defined set of rules that make up an unambiguous path, sometimes with branching structure, to guide a program or user to a logical endpoint. Alternative paths in the algorithm at branch points are taken on the basis of answers or conditions present at the steps before the branches. **Algorithms are also called "protocols," which are excellent when traversed by dedicated slave-like machines but useless when not traversed at all by humans.**

amoeba: The British spelling of ameba, which I like because it is more arcane, describing a general form of protozoan animals (single-celled) that move about and capture prey by gradually extending out temporary extensions of their cytoplasm called pseudopods and then "flowing" in that direction. They do not possess *cilia* or *flagella* to aid in movement.

analog: A term referring to signals that are "continuous" or to information that possesses an infinite number of gradations. Sound, for example, is a continuous wave of energy with varying frequencies, and there are an infinite number of possible points along the wave. Because this is reflective of actual life situations, it is called analog (analogous to real). If this continuous analog sound wave were to broken into 100 pieces and the frequency within each puzzle piece were sampled, the process of "digitization" would have been started. Each little puzzle piece could be converted into a specified number of *bits* or *bytes* to represent its sample characteristic, thus becoming data that the computer can manipulate. If the computer then takes the digitized bytes, reassembles them in sequence, and vocalizes them with a *sound* card, the resultant wave is very similar, although not identical, to the analog one initially sampled. The smaller, more numerous, and more compact the digital samples, the more closely the digital wave resembles the analog one. This same process can be applied to the colors or densities or degree of grayness of a visual image. The digital data can be transmitted over communications *media* and reassembled into sounds or images resembling the analog parent by computers at the other end.

API: (see application programming interface)

application: A software program specifically aimed at the user for the purpose of accomplishing a task. Examples are WordPerfect for text processing, Excel or Lotus for spreadsheets, and DOOM2 for mayhem.

application programming interface (API): The source code calling conventions by which an application program accesses operating software or other services. APIs can also serve as translators between different code formats in one or both directions.

application support: Direct help with learning, trouble-shooting, confidence building, and skills enhancement in the production environment after introduction of a new information system.

architecture: (see information system architecture)

archiving: The act of moving immediately accessible data from a computer to a storage medium, such as magnetic tape or optical disc, because it has filled up the on-line capacity of the system. The archived data is still obtainable, just not in a convenient or timely fashion. **The need for archived data rises exponentially just after roll-out has occurred, causing rancor among the user troops and forcing costly upgrades to computer storage capacity. After the expenditure, it plummets precipitately.**

artificial intelligence (AI): The label given when an inanimate machine makes a decision to take action independent of the cognitive intention of the human user. Also called decision support, because it requires the element of decision to differentiate it from the millions of other automatic actions computers take. **Whereas it is assumed that human brain activity always reflects decision making, and hence natural (free range) intelligence, this dignity cannot be bestowed on computers, which require artificial programming and rules to carry out beneficial processes. Developers are fond of exploiting this fact by**

displaying user error messages declaring: "I would like to take you seriously, but to do so would affront your intelligence."[3]

ASCII: Acronym for American National Standard Code for Information Interchange, which uses a coded character set consisting of 7-bit coded characters, 8 bits including parity check. **It is 100 percent accurate except that it sometimes omits the "N" character.**

Asymmetric Digital Subscriber Line, (ASDL): A technology developed to transmit video on demand over broadband copper wire communication media. Speed is 6 megabits/second downstream and 64 kilobits/second on return path. Newer symmetric digital subscriber line (SSDL) technology is emerging with even greater transmission speeds of nearly 2 megabits/second bidirectionally.

Asynchronous Transfer Mode, (ATM): Technology related to the simultaneous transmission of voice, video, and data at speeds up to hundreds of megabytes per second (faster than Ethernet LAN). Because it is rooted in international standards, it is likely to be a key enabler for telemedicine, wherein remote video (including endoscopy or other clinical images) can be guided and interpreted by specialists at geographically different sites in real time.

ATP: Adenosine triphosphate, the energy carrier molecule ADP (see above) with its third phosphate group, in which form it is ready to donate the energy from the third phosphate group bonds to facilitate an enzymatic transition step in a metabolic pathway. It directly or indirectly transfers energy to nearly all metabolic pathways, from photosynthesis in plants to life processes in animals. It consists of adenine (a base element of DNA), a simple sugar (ribose), and three phosphate groups. In its configuration with only two phosphate groups, it is called ADP, and, when it contains only one phosphate group, it is called AMP, in which case it functions as one of the most powerful and ubiquitous of chemical messengers. **Nature doesn't waste anything, and neither should management.**

authentication: The process a system employs to match an identified user to another piece of information (password, biometric) to ensure that they are valid individuals with user privileges.

availability: Refers to the amount of time a system, program, or network is available for use. Often described in days by hours (7 by 24). **In integration efforts, this can be meaningless, because, even if the unifying system is up 7 by 24, any one or several of the integrated systems could be down at any time.**

B

back-up: The process of making a copy of the files or programs on the hard disk and storing them in a physically different place than the main storage site, a form of *redundancy*. Back-ups of data on the hard disk should be made to floppy disks, magnetic tapes, or optical discs in order to avoid *disaster*. **Disaster is commonly perceived by novices to computer technology as the immediate natural reaction to any kind of change.**

bandwidth: A term referring to the range of frequencies a device or communication medium is capable of carrying. The greater the bandwidth, the higher the capacity of the line to handle larger and more diverse types of data.

baseband: A term used to describe a kind of communication medium that transmits only one channel of data.

baseline document: A chart of every single function, feature, computer screen, code path, and data object compiled and reproduced in microscopic font for all project team members; it serves as the absolute arbiter of what is in or out of scope. The baseline document will guide the production of *PCRs* and will constrain any creativity on the part of workers so that the sponsors of the effort will not lose faith in the project. Midway through a large development effort, when *scope creep* is at a peak and morale at a trough, managers get things back on track by mandating creation of project baseline documents. **Despite the fact that schedules have slipped like a Teflon sole on bat guano, and the financial status of things is less hopeful than the stock market on Black Tuesday, all energy is directed at reviewing the SOW and combing through design documents. The greatest utility of the baseline document, however, is that it points out where new functions need to be added and where critical omissions have occurred, thereby adding complexity and expense without really creeping scope.**

baud: Strictly speaking, the number of times an electronic signal can switch states in one second. More commonly, it refers to a unit of measure of data transmission between systems, defined as the number of bits of information that can cross a line per second. Named after a late 19th Century French telegraph operator named Baudot, who developed a five-bit coding system. **The bit, however, was not named after Bidet. Bauds are to modems as horsepower is to automobiles; you can never use all the horsepower on a racing machine to travel existing roads, and you can never fully flex your bauds on the current information highway. Still, it's not what you can really do, but how you look that counts.**

big bang: The name of the all-at-once approach to implementing a new system. Advisable in some situations and treacherous in others, depending on user readiness and the degree of operational change and *infobia* associated with the system.

bio-enterprise framework: A new method of visualizing and categorizing enterprise structure based on general classes of living animals, which takes into account the important role of information and emphasizes concepts of cooperation, messaging, specialization, and real-time monitoring of factors effecting *homeostasis*. The four models within the framework are the single-celled *protozoan*, the multicelled sponge, the *simple animal* (with nervous system), and the *complex animal* (utilizing hormones and a circulatory system).

biometrics: Refers to physical characteristics of users (fingerprints, handprints, voiceprints, retinal scans, iris traits, etc.) that systems store and use to authenticate identity before allowing user access to a system. **It is also the enormously boring statistical study of biological entities, sometimes taught during medical school.**

bio-transition framework: The application of the biological/meta-bolic change process to transitions within enterprises, emphasizing the roles of resistance (activation energy), change agents (enzymes), and management discipline (energy carriers) in the successful implementation of change in organizations.

bit: Computers process data in binary form, meaning they understand only if single electrical units are on or off. Because there are only two choices, on or off, the unit of data in a binary system can have only two digits: 0 or 1. Thus, the unit of data is a binary digit, a bit. These bits are pretty small, so it takes a number of them in a bunch to encode one character of information. This package, which is treated as a single unit by the computer, is called a byte. **All computerized data and information can be blown to bits.**

blob (binary large object): A fantastic new object-oriented data structure that gathers a miraculous number of data attributes into one convenient place. Blobs are not interpreted by the primary database system, but can be deciphered with other tools. This feature is one that analysts have been dreaming of for years, because it coalesces logically related elements into a form that is perfect for scientific or business studies. **As futuristic as the Starship Enterprise, the blob structure has another Trekian trait: it completely cloaks its valuable elements from view by anyone but the database designers.**

BOFIB: Acronym for bigger or faster is better, also called Rose's acronym.

boot: The process a computer goes through when powered up, in which it awakens, initiates its *operating system* software, monitors its resources and *peripherals*, and steels itself for your commands. "Cold boot" occurs when the computer has been without power and is switched on; "warm boot" (also called "reboot") occurs when the booting procedure is invoked during a session by depressing the Ctrl-Alt-Del keys on the keyboard simultaneously, allowing a fresh start after a crash. **Ctrl-Alt-Del is the most frequently recorded keystroke combination.**

bottleneck: A term describing any of a multitude of points or individuals in a development process at which there is no possibility of adding resources to speed progress. Frequently applied to an individual with critical expertise on a project who cannot possibly work any harder or longer without decompensating, it can also be applied to blockages in program performance or database execution. **Also a term used to refer to the curious physical appearance of some developers, used in association with the related terms "geek" and "stooge." Bottleneck individuals should not be openly identified lest they inflate their sense of self-worth and demand more compensation.**

bridge: A device similar to a router that is used to connect different kinds of *communications media* to the computers on a network. It passes "packets" of bits from one network to another. Bridges make teleconferencing possible (simultaneous communication). Bridges on steroids, called multipoint conferencing units (MCUs), are the culprits that enabled *video conferencing*, with sound and video transmission.

broadband: A term used to describe a kind of communications medium that can transmit multiple channels of data simultaneously.

bugs: Little idiosyncrasies in software that disallow smooth application function. The term seems to have originated among telegraph operators in America's first "high technology" system, who discussed the insects cohabiting their workplaces. Thomas Edison used the term in 1878 to describe little faults or difficulties that required intense study prior to commercial success—or failure.[4] **Bugs are different from defects, in that they are not always the result of programming errors, but rather represent spontaneous mutations in the code. They are an inevitable force of nature. Bugs often masquerade as "features." It is believed that evolution of bugs gave rise to more advanced computer organisms, such as worms and even mice.**

build: The process of converting software code written by humans in a higher level *programming language* (such as C or C++) into specific machine-level modules containing operational steps in the form of binary messages. The conversion is done by a software program called a *compiler*. **Somewhat contrary to the English usage notion that build means to construct or put something together, a code build means to pulverize it into atomic parts and store it for use. "We are having a problem with the build" is one of the most frequent utterances of developers.**

byte: A grouping of bits that encode one character of information, which is treated as a single unit by the computer. A page of double-spaced text contains about a thousand bytes of information, and, because the metric system is generally applied in computer systems, this would be one kilobyte of information. (actually there turn out to be 1,024 bytes in a kilobyte, and, trust me, you don't want to know why). A thousand of these kilobytes are referred to as a megabyte, and a thousand megabytes are referred to as a gigabyte. **These bytes are important in impressing others with your hardware, because the size of one's hard disk, though not everything, is a fundamental part of self-esteem. The average floppy disk measures about 2-3 megabytes.**

C

call-back: A method for increasing the security of systems being accessed by *modems*. The initial user contact over the phone line is into a modem, or a *router*, which presents security log-on screens and requests a *password*. The router then disconnects the caller, looks up the authorized phone number of the identified user, and dials the modem back, again asking for a password and then allowing access to the system.

can: The term used to connote the container in which you put software that has undergone all of its testing and is awaiting delivery to the production environment. **It may be the same receptacle into which you place the software after delivery to the production environment if you fail with implementation.**

catalyst: A substance, usually used in small amounts relative to reactants, that modifies and increases the rate of a reaction without being consumed in the process. In living processes, these are enzymes, and they act by diminishing the activation energy required to achieve the critical transition state necessary for a change to occur. In the business sense, catalysts can be viewed as change agents who facilitate a process or event without being changed or destroyed in the process. Using various communication, interpersonal, and managerial techniques, change agents lower the transition energy necessary to implement a business process change.

CD/CD-ROM: Abbreviations for compact disc (CD, optical disc) and Compact Disc, Read Only Memory. These are plastic disks pitted with laser readable dips and coated with aluminum and lacquer as opposed to magnetic substances. They can hold large amounts of information (up to 6 gigabytes). The most common of these is the CD-ROM, which can be read by but not written to by the computer and which is usually accessed through the D: drive. This is the same technology used in music CDs, holding in the range of 660 megabytes of data. CD-ROM playback rates are indicated as 2X, 4X, up to 12X currently. BOFIB.

cell: The basic living unit capable of "living" independently and reproducing, given appropriate resources and conditions. It basically consists of a nucleus, cytoplasm, and a cell membrane, all of which function together to maintain balance with internal conditions and environmental circumstances. Also a term used to refer to a small unit of resources (users, nodes, computers, or services) that work together and are administered together. In the distributed computing environment, this means that the cell has its own separately administered communications, directories, security, and time servers. **The cell in DCE can rightly be referred to as a "padded cell.'**

cell membrane: A double molecular layer of fat (lipids) that serves as a selective barrier between the fluids inside a cell and the environment outside the cell. *Proteins* are embedded in the lipid layer and carry out membrane regulatory and sensation functions. Their key role is to balance concentration and amounts of water and chemicals between the *cytoplasm* and the outside world.

central data repository (CDR): A term for a single logical or physical container of data collected from or to be delivered to peripheral servers or systems. Sometimes abstrusely called a data warehouse, the CDR is relatively easy and pleasurable to conceive, but painful and difficult to deliver. **The efforts involved in the actual creation of a CDR have been likened to those of a one-legged cat trying to bury scat on a frozen pond.**

central processing unit (CPU): That part of a computing system containing the micro-electronic circuits and microprocessors (chips) that actually interpret and execute *software* instructions and carry out complex arithmetic and logical computations via electron cascades that result in actions. The chips and micro-electronics elements are fastened to a fiberglass board or card; the main circuits are on the *motherboard*, also called the logic board. CPUs were given chip class numbers and letter designations in ancient times (e.g., 386DX or 386SX), but, since the introduction of Intel's Pentium, chips have been rated by the speed with which they process information, measured in megahertz (MHz, thousand cycles per second). The larger the number, the faster the chip and the more expensive the machine. **(One should ignore the fact that humans can't really detect any enhancement of performance over about 120 MHz for the vast majority of applications and buy the fastest chip available. Owning a non-Pentium chip is a valid reason to whine, complain, and upgrade.)**

CGI: (see common gateway interface)

change agents: Business catalysts who facilitate a process or event, without being changed or destroyed in the process. Using various communication, interpersonal, and managerial techniques, change agents lower the transition energy (effort), also called resistance, necessary to implement a business process change.

change control board (CCB): Once integration has been achieved between disparate systems through *interfaces* (in an attempt to create liberation within the information system environment), a CCB is convened to deal with the fact that the slightest change to one linked system has a very high probability of breaking all of the other related systems. **This group realizes that liberation is actually imprisonment and begins the ongoing task of managing the prisoners. If integration has not been achieved, the CCB can turn its attention to PCRs, wherein its chief function is to decide, after prolonged and heated discussion, to take issues off line for resolution.**

change management: A fascinating term in that it engenders strikingly common emotional effects in different groups, even though the groups have completely different understandings of what the term means. To the administators it incites panic at the thought of managing worker behavior, whereas in technologists it creates angst at the prospect of changing hardware, software, or processes that can destabilize an integrated system. **A similar phenomemon is observed with the utterance: "fire" whether in the board room, a theater, or a military engagement.**

change management consultants: Individuals with expertise in assessing and suggesting the best methods for walking into the whirling propellers of technological change in an established business environment. **These consultants often have degrees in sociology: the study of those who do not need to be studied by those who do.[5] These individuals are particularly helpful with computer applications in health care, where change has rarely been observed and where clinical experience, resulting from years of making the same mistakes over and over, is sanctified.**

cilia: Plural of cilium, referring to short, hair-like extensions of a cell membrane, containing microtubules that facilitate their motion. Cilia are typically multiple and serve to propel an organism, move fluid around the cell, or act as part of sensory structures.

client-server: A type of *information system architecture* in which larger computers (servers) send information to smaller computers (clients). A single computer can function as a client and a server. Both of the connected computers must have *CPUs* (i.e., neither is a dumb terminal, which is nothing more than a keyboard and a monitor).

clone: A computer that functions in a manner similar to one manufactured by another company, capable of running the same programs and having the same *platform*. Also, an exact replica or copy or programs and configuration parameters made from one server for rapid installation on another server. **If one cloned a sheep and emerged with a heifer, an approximate simulation of the results of server cloning would have been attained. Also refers to any number of computers available by mail order at extraordinarily good prices, which can be used to undermine the business rewards of the company that really deserves the credit for original work.**

code: *Software* instructions created using *programming language* to induce computer processes that support the functional requirements set forth in the external and internal design documents. The core activity of system development.

code push: Transmission of a software program or application update from a central site to other computers over a network, as opposed to actually walking over to the computers and loading software onto them in person. (The latter approach is called "sneaker net.")

commensalism: Long-term interaction between two species in which one species benefits significantly while the other is neither helped nor harmed significantly.

common gateway interface (CGI): A set of Internet-based interface programs that allow information entered by a user on web pages to be seen on the Internet server, or vice versa.

common systems: A term used to describe the situation in which an enterprise or series of linked operations all use the same information system to carry out their business. In fact, common systems are mostly a myth; even well-conceived identical systems deployed in differing environments remain common for a matter of milliseconds before local information system departments make code changes to suit specific provincial operations needs.

communications media: Refers to the kind of substance or method used to connect hardware devices, examples being copper wire; coaxial cable; fiberoptic cable; and radio-frequency waves, infrared waves, and microwaves.

compatible software: Software written in a way that it can be executed on a particular piece of computer hardware. Applications written for Apple computers using MacIntosh operating systems may not be compatible with IBM PCs using Windows or OS2 operating systems (see platform). Some software can be run on multiple different platforms (and is therefore called a "cross-platform" application). Other programs must be converted, or "ported," onto different platforms if they are to be executable.

compiler: A software program that is employed during a *build* of code to translate high-level *programming language* into machine language that

computer microprocessors can use directly as instructions. **The importance of a compiler stems from its common English definition: a col-
lector of words, a lexicographer, a connoisseur, a dilettante, a person
of taste, a linguist.**

complex animal: A model in the bio-enterprise framework representing a very highly integrated and specialized organization that is heavily
reliant on multiple kinds of information systems, the most notable of
which is the free-flow dissemination of messages that act like hormones,
causing precise specific or global responses in sensitive targets.

compoacher: A term I made up to refer to someone who steals, defiles,
or breeches the security of others' computer systems. The term is derived
from the obsolete French pocher: to poke, thrust, or intrude. It should be
used in place of *hacker*, which is an inappropriate term to use when referring to these criminals.

component: A set of armor-plated objects that interface with one
another in object-oriented programs.

component object model (COM): The technical underpinning of
Microsoft's *OLE*, which facilitates handling objects over a network.

computer: A machine that accepts data input, processes that data in a
defined manner, and presents the results of the processing in a fashion
that is comprehensible to the user. The elements of the computer that
can be broken with a hammer are called "hardware." The invisible
instructions that direct the hardware are called "software." Software that
enables a set of useful activities may also be referred to as an "application." The largest computers are called "mainframes," and the smaller
and more familiar ones are called personal computers. In fact, the practice of categorizing computers by size has become absurd, because anything that takes data in, processes it and puts data out is a computer,
regardless of size or power. **The computer is often mistaken as a solution for business problems and is frequently blamed for failure,
when, in fact, human behavior is the root of the evil. They do, however, make inhumanely fast, incredibly accurate errors.**

computer-based training (CBT)*:* A technique using the multimedia
capabilities of computers to deliver interactive training to users who can
be directed by tutorial on use of a new application while actually exercis-
ing it on line. A very stable application is required to develop CBT, and
the development of CBT is relatively expensive, but retention from such
training is usually high, and, if an application is to be used for a high user
volume over a long period without significant changes, it may be very
effective. **It is also lonely, boring, and tedious and can be offensive to
those with high degrees of initial infobia.**

configuration management system (CMS) document: This document provides written instructions detailing exactly what kinds of hardware are needed to run a application, and how to load, unload, *boot*,
reboot, take down, *back-up*, and solve problems in a system. It elucidates
steps for monitoring operations and recovering lost *files*, as well as for
determining when *CPU* power is outgrown or disc space is inadequate.
Perhaps the most important document in information systems

departments, the CMS is critical to keeping things limping along as programmer after programmer leaves the operation.

confirm step: A point in project development methodology after system and integration testing but before user acceptance testing wherein the functions of the application are demonstrated to the customer in order to convince buyers that the code is grossly in line with expectations. **Generally a happy time in a project, preceding the explosion of bugs, defects, issues, and miserable performance that will be revealed in user acceptance testing.**

Conservation of User Energy Principle (COUEP): Any change users must make to utilize new technology will require energy (and probably time) and the initial energy expended must be recaptured in a relatively immediate fashion from the technology if the users are to have any likelihood of continuing with the process. If there is not an overall time/comfort savings resulting from the new technology, change will not occur or will not persist.

consolidation: From the Latin *consolidatus*, meaning "to make firm," this refers to the process of uniting individual design elements into a coherent whole. It implies the production of a uniform, well-digested, well-formed product. **The opposite of consoliflatus.**

consultants: Individuals of varying abilities and motivations who are called in to give advice and provide direction when organizations perceive the need for outside expertise in an area. (Consultants often lack expertise in the area, but their association with management gives t' illusion that any bad decisions that get made are not solely the respon bility of executives, and it is this "scapegoat" function that allows ex, . tion of exorbitant consultation fees. Sometimes consultants give advic that should be passed on to competitors rather than used directly, and other times the statement of the obvious is exactly what an enterprise needs (see *change management consultants*). Because advice giving is generally offensive (except for that given in this book), the diplomacy of its delivery is often the key to consulting, and one should carefully evaluate the tact and style of the messenger in selecting what could easily develop into commensalism with the enterprise.

contingency funding: A small amount of money (usually less than 10 percent of a project's budget) that is set aside for unanticipated needs during the project life cycle. **These funds are also referred to as "starter bucks," as they are often spent immediately. In some cases, it is wise to avoid budgeting contingency funds in order to give project managers a maximum amount of anxiety from the get go and to give those funding the work the necessary false sense that everyone has clearly thought through every detail of the project.**

convergence: A term implying moving toward standard data definitions, terminology, and coding schemes and convergence on standards of communications such that information can be shared and compared, regardless, of where, how, or on what platform it is derived. Sometimes misused to imply that every related enterprise should work toward the same information platform or technology solution.

cooperative development: A process wherein developers or business and technical partners with a common vision attempt to work in parallel toward a goal. The hope is that, by not duplicating efforts or products and by lending special domain expertise, more will be accomplished faster. **Numerous large- and small-scale experiments have consistently proved with statistically valid scientific evidence that cooperative development is impossible because it is completely inconsistent with human nature. Work is ongoing, however.**

CORBA (common object request broker architecture): Similar to OLE, a component technology for handling objects over a network from various distributed platforms.

core dump: A common nongastrointestinal evacuation of important data from a large database, generally occurring after several hours of toil on a system. **Often confused with a sister term, cor zero, which is the situation that occurs when all cardiac activity ceases in the developer who has irrevocably lost work as a result of the dump.**

cost/benefit evaluation: One of the most troubling and difficult concepts in management, particularly in the realm of information systems (because they are so expensive), this refers to the balance of the cost of acquisition of a system and its predicted economic benefits. This is a quantitative assessment that is often used to guide strategic decisions about company expenditures. Sometimes referred to as a "return on investment" analysis. Even when a valid cost/benefit study is achieved in the area of information systems, economic benefits are often not realized, because the critical follow-up process of harvesting the savings is much more difficult than predicting them. **When blindly examining the cost/benefit elephant, almost everyone seizes the tail and is soon steeped in controversy.**

cost/effectiveness evaluation: The gifted sibling of cost/benefit evaluation, this is an evaluation of the cost of acquisition of a system vis-à-vis its effects on the organization in total, which is much more qualitative, and therefore real, but immeasurable. Most of the systems that users want cannot be proved cost-beneficial, but they are intuitively cost-effective. The process of converting qualitative items (i.e., better communication, improved access to information, better decision making, higher quality, fewer wasteful activities) into value equivalents requires expert opinion, usually by management engineers or, for the less fortunate, consultants. **After time-motion studies, flow structure diagrams, on-sight observation, and extensive interviews, usually at great expense, consultants and engineers can turn the ethereal organizational benefits into favorable numbers just long enough to persuade steering committees of the strategic advantage of a system.**

COUEP: (see conservation of user energy principle)

CPU: (see central processing unit)

crash: One of two kinds of problems that occur when running a computer application. The less concerning of these is also called a "hose," "bomb," or "lockup," which is really an *ABEND*, wherein a program is prematurely ceased and not recoverable short of starting over. The second and worse of the two problems is a "head" or "hard disk" crash, wherein the reading device (head) of the drive malfunctions and impales itself on the disk, obliterating the *bytes* that are stored there and generally causing an irretrievable loss of data (*disaster*).

critical enabler: An indispensable substance, process, or infrastructural element needed to traverse a pathway or to accomplish a business process. Sometimes, enabler is reserved for applications that have value on the road to greater efficiency or productivity but that have little intrinsic cost-benefit in and of themselves. Information systems often fit this category.

critical pathway: A series of events in the development of a system solution, the successful completion of which is judged to be essential to proceeding any further (see project plan and progress). This term can properly apply to any and every pathway in an integrated project. **Multiple critical pathways may converge at a critical angle on a critical point. If this happens rapidly, critical velocity is achieved, leading to critical mass and therefore a critical state, wherein critical pressure is exerted, leaving the project in critical condition.**

critical success factor: Anything that must go as expected in order for a project or organization to achieve a goal. It does not mean that success is ensured if the critical success factor is maintained, however, as has been repeatedly demonstrated. **Often about as relevant as Pavarotti's diet plan.**

CRUD diagram: A complex matrix relating business functions and subject areas to all other function and subject areas based on whether users in the areas create, read, update, or delete data, hoping to show data dependencies.

cytoplasm: The cellular parts, fluids, and substances enclosed by the *cell membrane*, except the *nucleus*.

D

daemon: A very aptly named bit of software chicanery wherein a process is initiated automatically in the code, without user intervention or choice. **Daemons allow developers to avoid the hours of thought necessary to intelligently design a process.**

data dictionary: A list of data elements, structures, and models with their relationships and attributes, using standard naming conventions and demonstrating their relationship to business entities.

data element: The smallest logical scrap of data.

data model: Sometimes called a data structure or a data object, data models comprise data elements and attributes related to business entities.

data structure: A grouping of data elements that, by virtue of their proximity, can be associated with an *entity*.

data validity: The assurance that a datum or set of data is accurate, not corrupted or incorrect.

database: A set or collection of information stored in one of several forms on a computer. Flat-file databases allow users to work with only one data table or set of fields at a time, whereas relational databases (Sybase, Oracle) allow multiple tables or sets of fields to be worked with at the same time. A new type of database, called "object-oriented," manages concepts with multiple attributes and relationships to other objects (see *knowledge base*), having evolved dramatically from the concept of tables.

DCE (distributed computing environment): An extraordinary set of software that has become a de facto standard for managing and administering client server computing environments. It is a very complex "middleware" program (hidden from end users) that has major components: Remote procedure call (RPC), which allows individual parts of an application to run on computers elsewhere in a network; security services (no cool acronym), which manages distributed security registries, authentication parameters, and user privileges; directory services (also called cell directory services, CDS), which is used to locate users, computers, applications, and printers on a network; distributed time service (DTS), which provides clock synchronization between computers on a network; and a whole bunch of other stuff that seeks (almost successfully) to provide the beautiful organization and the balance of multiple simultaneous diverse processes that occur in living organisms. **The client server equivalent of metabolism.**

debugging: The steps taken to identify, locate, and repair code anomalies that prevent proper software operation. There are programs called debuggers that can aid in this otherwise labor-intensive process, but one must realize that, even after a bug fix, all of the *testing* must be repeated to be sure that the software repair has not created new *defects*. **Debuggers are software applications as well, and a very delicate situation develops when they have bugs; the flea on a fly syndrome.**

default: Another unique information system term with meaning antonymous to regular English use. Whereas the populous believes that default means to fail to meet an obligation, information specialists know that a default is an ensured action that the application unfailingly performs as directed by the user or the system.

defect (severity levels): A failure of *software* to perform as required by *external* and *internal design documents*. Best tracked with scientific notation, defects are programming errors that are revealed by *test scripts*. Two fascinating defect varieties are "intermittent defects," which occur only under some circumstances or in specific environments (and therefore don't have to be revealed to users) and "upstream" defects, which block testers from further code exploration. The latter is like a dam; it must be fixed quickly so that testers can hurtle uncontrollably over the plunging rapids beyond. **Defects are graded by severity. Severity one: The system completely crashes because of the defect. Severity two: The system suffers miserably, struggles in agony, gasps, and causes interfaced systems to crump without completely hosing, and there is no workaround. Severity three: The system works in an aberrant fashion, requiring extreme workaround measures on the part of testers or**

users to circumvent the defect. **This is considered to be successful code. Severity four: Misspellings, screen inconsistencies, data errors, and style gaffes that make users pine for a severity one defect.**

deliverable: Items promised to customers are loosely referred to as deliverables. Most deliverables are detailed in the *SOW*. Examples of deliverables in addition to the software itself might include design or *CMS* documents, user guides, training manuals, and even support personnel. **When promises for goods or services must be forcefully extracted, they are referred to as "forceps deliverables"; when they are produced out of order, they are "breech deliverables"; and when they are turned over before they have been completely finished, they are "premature deliverables."**

design documents: Written records of project requirements and intentions. There are several types. Joint application design document (JAD) is notes from sessions with users solidifying a set of essential design elements that are guaranteed to be outside the scope of the project as planned. These serve as a basis for crafting the internal and external design documents.

desk-top: The name given to the opening *graphical user interface* display on a computer screen, containing an array of program and file *icons*. One can "arrange" one's desk-top, change its colors and print styles, and decorate it with picturesque backgrounds, which is the first pleasurable activity generally undertaken by a new user. **Usually, a politically incorrect background is selected.**

developer: Refers to an individual who writes software code in a language that can be compiled and loaded on a computer. Developers are charged with the enormous responsibility of converting user needs into computer actions. **They generally deliver systems that increase cost, decrease efficiency, and add complexity to daily activities. Also term employed by users as a synonym for idiot (see reciprocal context at user).**

development methodology: A prescribed series of steps or principles to be followed from embarkation on a project to delivery of product, elucidating the path of iteration, development, testing, piloting, acceptance, etc. Fundamental to the project plan, development methodology is intended to be relatively simple. **If it succeeds in being simple and understandable, it will necessarily be inadequate.**

digital versatile disc (DVD): The next generation of compact discs can store up to 14 times more information than current CDs and can play it back at a rate of 11 million bits per second. (This rate is equivalent to a 9X CD-ROM capability.) DVDs are pitted on two surfaces, and the pits are half the size of those on current CDs, yielding a data spiral that is 11 kilometers long. Using new formatting technology, DVDs allow recording of more information per pit, and, combined with technology that actually layers pit surfaces, storage of more than 17 gigabytes of data per disc is quite feasible. This means one DVD not only can hold an entire movie, but also could store different languages of dialogue, different cuts and camera angles, and ultimately Dolby-type, theater quality sound encoding.[6]

digital: Refers to information represented as discreet values consisting of binary messages (on or off, *bits* or *bytes*). Continuous or infinite entities, called *analog,* can be sampled in pieces and converted to digital messages that are the only kind a computer can manipulate. Digitized information samplings can be reassembled into articles that very closely represent the original analog entity.

disaster: Any event that destroys or disables computer files or programs. Disasters can be major, such as occur in acts of God (hurricanes, earthquakes, spontaneous combustion), or less major, as occur with acts of humans (coke spillage, static electricity, gum). Sometimes the data can be recovered, and this process is called disaster recovery. Prevention of disaster is always better than disaster recovery, and so data are often duplicated (also called *redundancy*) and stored at a site remote from the main operation. **Disaster is a term also applied to roll-out. Even after a successful roll-out, disaster can be claimed if a competitive product is more successful than your own.**

disaster recovery: Specific procedures for restoring or recovering data and information that may have been damaged or disabled by a disaster. Also used to refer to restoring availability of a system that has gone down, which, in the eyes of the user, is a disaster.

disconnect: The name given to the sudden realization that there is no common understanding whatsoever between customers and developers about an element of an application. Often, a disconnect can be shown to have been previously evaluated, detailed, documented, and communicated. **If scope creep is the spreading toe fungus of a project, disconnects are the accompanying foot odor. Everyone is advised to keep their shoes on.**

disintermediation: A term referring to the desirable situation in which a computer information system or operational change obviates the need for wasteful human activities, thereby allowing a reduction in staff, improved efficiency, avoidance of cost, and justification for undertaking automation or *reengineering.* **Usually the disintermediated position will require replacement by two more expensive, highly trained scarce individuals.**

disk: Any of several thin cylindrical objects coated with substances that can record strings of binary (off-on) electronic indicators (*bits*). Hard disk: rigid plastic disks (there are commonly several of these stacked together) with magnesium oxide coating that reside permanently within the computer housing, used as the primary medium to present programs and receive data. Usually located in the C: drive, hard drives have a relatively high information storage capacity (500 megabytes-5 gigabytes). Floppy disk: more pliable plastic discs, coated in the same fashion as hard disks, that can store information or programs to be accessed when inserted into the slot of the A: drive of most computers. These come in two sizes (3.5 and 5.25 inch diameter) and hold much less information than a hard disk (1.4-2.8 megabytes). Compact disc (CD, optical disc): plastic disks pitted with laser readable dips and coated with aluminum and lacquer as opposed to magnetic substances. They can hold large amounts of information (up to 6 gigabytes). The most common disk is the CD-ROM (Compact Disc, Read Only Memory), which can be read by but not written to by the computer and which is usually accessed through the D: drive. This is the same technology used in music CDs, holding in the range of 660 megabytes of data. CD-ROM playback rates are indicated as 2X, 4X, or 6X currently. BOFIB. Digital Versatile Discs (DVD): the next generation of compact discs can store up to 14 times more information than current CDs and can play it back at a rate of 11 million bits per second.

distributed component object model (DCOM): The form of COM (component object model) technology that enables handling of objects over a network.

document: Any of a number of "papers" illuminating project elements. The EDR (external design report) is a formal, detailed, extensive, analytic narrative documenting precise requirements for design and development of a function in a complex computer application (containing an undetectable disastrous mistake. The Internal design report *IDR is a* detailed document similar to the external design document but distinguished from the former in that it focuses entirely on elements of the system's internal functions **in technically indecipherable language, ignoring the external design requirements, and containing more than one undetectable disastrous mistake.**

documentation: A term used to describe many types of written material generated in a system development or implementation effort: design, system, configuration management, and baseline documents are examples.

DOS: A kind of operating system software, originally developed by Microsoft (MS-DOS), reinvented by IBM (PC-DOS), and adopted by several others, that does not have a graphical user interface. **If you are a new computer user, you do not want DOS. If you are an experienced computer user, you aren't reading this definition.**

download: To obtain software or data from another computer over communications media. **Downloaded programs can be shareware or freeware, or virus-laden executable files that give your computer horrible sores.**

dual systems: The uncomfortable and expensive process of running an old system or process in parallel with a new one during implementation of the new one, because everyone really needs to be on a single system for adequate business delivery. In this case, the old system remains the de facto standard until the new one is completely rolled out, which requires duplication of efforts in most cases and which is why rapid roll-out is preferable whenever possible.

due diligence: The actions associated with making a good decision. These actions include investigation of legal, technical, human, and financial predictions and of the ramifications of proposed enterprise endeavors, particularly when a partner or vendor is to be involved.

Duh's Principle: A point of saturation will be reached on a project at which the addition of qualified, energetic new individuals with superb work ethics and great attitudes will have an overall damaging effect on progress. A difficult principle to grasp, it assumes that all project members are qualified, energetic individuals with superb work ethics and great attitudes and that the time needed to bring a new member up to speed would only put the project further behind. **Duh's Principle is invoked any time someone really good comes along (to protect incompetents) and every time the budget ceiling has been reached.**

dumb terminal: A computer screen (monitor) and keyboard, without a CPU. Dumb terminals cannot run programs in and of themselves but can be used as extensions of a mainframe computer to manipulate *software* on the host.

DVD: (see Digital Versatile Discs)

E

education: For the purposes of this book, education is the process of constant communication of values, reasons, and methods for changing to any individuals who will be affected by the change in or around a business. It involves managing *infobia*, as well as *training* and development of an environment of trust and integrity.

effector: In living systems, a tissue or target organ that responds to nerve transmissions by inducing motion or changes in internal conditions that aid in the maintenance of *homeostasis*. A key differentiator of the sponge model from the *simple animal* model in the *bio-enterprise framework*.

enabler: Some substance, process, or infrastructural element needed to to traverse a pathway or accomplish a business process. Sometimes, enabler is reserved for applications that have value on the road to greater efficiency or productivity but that have little intrinsic cost-benefit in and of themselves. Information systems often fit this category.

encryption: The process of transforming free text (also called clear text) into cypher-text, which is essentially an unintelligible string of characters and symbols. This encrypted data can be transmitted over communications media with a high degree of security and then decrypted (deciphered) when it reaches its secure destination.

encryption key: An element of an encryption algorithm, such as a password, that must be supplied by a user to enable the encryption transformation to occur.

end product: The result of a step in a transformation, or in a series of transformations.

end-game: A term applied to the ideal state, when desired application functions are complete and performing flawlessly. The product of excellent *project vision*. **Synonymous with Nirvana, miraculous, utopia, impossible.**

endocrine system: The complex set of glands and nerves that secrete hormones, which influence the activities of target tissues and cells.

energy: The capacity to do work, the effort to make things happen or change from one state to another, or what must be expended to keep homeostatic balance and defy entropy.

energy carrier: Molecules that are capable of storing or providing energy, in the presence of enzymes, that enables transitions in a metabolic pathway. *ATP/ADP* are the primary energy carriers in virtually all living systems.

energy state diagram: A graph depicting change in energy versus time as reactants undergo transformation to end products. The key elements are the beginning energy state, the ending energy state, and the activation energy required to get the reactants to a transition state (over the hill).

enterprise model: The diagram or definition of an aggregate of organization *entities* and their relationships, describing the very essence of the core business, independent of organizational structure. Until one understands the relevant enterprise model, one cannot design or develop useful computer applications to advance an organization toward it goals. The more complex an enterprise, or the more poorly understood the processes, the more likely it will be that automation attempts will fail. From the Old French "entreprendre," to undertake. (Also the origin of "undertaker.")

entity: An item (conceptual or real) that an organization needs in order to manage production of service delivery. Its related *data structure* is therefore something a business would like to measure, record, or manipulate using an information system. Entities are interrelated, and can be diagrammed, modeled, decomposed, aggregated, and typed. **Isolation and description of an entity requires efforts of the same magnitude as those expended to discover the mu meson in the nucleus of atomic particles.**

entropy: Basically speaking, the natural tendency of everything to tend toward disorder and randomness within a system. In living systems, it is the general measure of low-quality energy (generally heat) in the system that is so randomly dispersed as to be unavailable to do work. Homeostasis is the sum of the energy and processes necessary to keep the organism from the natural physical tendency of everything to disperse.

environment: The combination of hardware, network, and protocols that constitute the cyberworld in which the computer system functions. Problems with systems are generally attributed either to the code (software defects or bugs) or to the environment, (which implies that the code is perfect and the problems are with the network. **This is very convenient, in that it allows a flood of finger pointing when things are going poorly.**

enzyme: A special kind of *protein* with the ability to catalyze (speed) biological reactions in a metabolic pathway. It has very specific, three-dimensional active sites for the reactants, which it brings into proximity or stresses appropriately, thereby decreasing the activation energy normally required to induce a transition from substrate to end product. Enzymes catalyze reactions that would normally occur given enough time; they are extremely specific in their actions, are not altered in the course of facilitating the change, and can catalyze the reaction in either direction. Enzymes are analogous to change agents in business.

ergonomics: Consideration or applied science of configuring, designing, and arranging tools and environments that facilitate user efficiency, productivity, comfort, and safety.

Ethernet: A specific kind of *LAN* used within a building to connect computers and shared peripherals. It usually consists of coaxial cable (thick or thin) with a specific set of data communication protocols for sending, receiving, and sensing data. It transmits data in 64-byte packages with a maximum speed of 14,800 packets per second.

executable: A term that can be used to refer to the fact that a software module can be run (e.g., is executable) on a given *platform*. Such modules are often called "executables" and will contain a file name extension .exe. **The term also refers to valued project team members with extensive knowledge who are threatening to leave.**

F

facilitator: An individual in a meeting with the responsibility of guiding the discussion, monitoring progress, mediating conflict, reframing issues, clarifying observations, and managing egos, while at the same time remaining dispassionate and remote. Facilitators are sometimes not directly involved in project issues so that they can remain unbiased in their approach to the problems.

FAO: (see functional area owner)

fault tolerance: A term describing computer architecture that ensures maximum performance and minimal failure or downtime. Fault-tolerant systems generally require redundant storage media, power supply, and other critical components. **Also used to describe developers' unrealistic expectations that users of their systems will "tolerate" aberrations. The most accurate application of the term is to the immunity facilitators of a JAD session have to the peccadilloes and character pathology of those with whom they disagree.**

FDDI: (see Fiber Distributed Data Interface)

feature: A functional piece of a *software* application that can reasonably be viewed as a unit. If, for example, a computer screen resembles a prescription pad to be used to automatically order a medication, there might be a number of actions that could be invoked that would be features: specifying the medicine name, designating the pharmacy location to which the prescription is to be sent, or indicating that no generic drug is to be substituted for the trade medication ordered. In aggregate, features make up a "function" (prescription writing), which, in turn, is part of an application (order entry). A list of features is handy for tracking software *deliverables*. **Introduction of the list to the steering committee is called a feature presentation.**

feedback loops: The operation in which the products of a transition or transition process cause the process to be slowed (negative feedback) or speeded (positive feedback). Organisms sense conditions and use feedback loops to regulate activities. In business, the same types of loops can occur, the most effective of which is a positive feedback loop that is invoked when users recognize the benefits of an induced change and thus think creatively about additional methods for improving performance.

Fiber Distributed Data Interface (FDDI): The Schwarzenegger of LAN technology, FDDI uses fiberoptic cable to connect computers and devices. Also called a "backbone," the FDDI is often used to connect servers or LANs to each other. It can transmit a whopping 170,000 64-byte packages of data per second. Son of FDDI, FDDI-II, transmits data just as fast, but it can utilize copper wire as well as fiberoptic cable and can carry line voice and/or video data in addition to conventional packet data.

file: A collection of information stored in one convenient place for use by you and/or the computer. Files are generally of two major types: those that contain programs and those that contain data. Particularly large files are sometimes called directories, which are like hanging file folders into which you stuff multiple smaller files. **Like the "directory" during the French Revolution, computer directories are often riddled with corruption. Computerphile is a homonymous term meaning computer lover; the opposite is computerphobes (those fearing computers), who make up the majority of your work force.**

file transfer protocol (FTP): A protocol that allows a computer user to send data files to or receive data files from another computer over a TCP/IP network.

firewall: A set of security measures designed to protect internal information systems from abuse by outsiders who may be able to access your system through community networks (Internet). Any time a connection to the world wide web is established, a firewall should be erected to keep hackers from viewing, stealing, or corrupting data. **The ultimate firewall is to prohibit a connection completely. This is the approach that has been exploited by companies still using Morse code and carrier pigeons.**

flagella: Plural of flagellum, which is a modification of the cell membrane containing a microtubule system that generates motion. Often singular or sparse in number, they are similar to cilia, except they are often longer. They act to move the organism or to move fluid around the organism or cell.

flood: Incapacitating messages or unnecessary data transmission over a network that impede performance and communication. Also sometimes referred to as a storm. To experience it first hand, configure a TLS multitier distributed environment with the switches in front of the routers rather than with the routers attaching directly to the TLS. **If you heed the advice and avoid the flood, you can thank me for saving you thousands of hours and dollars trying to make things work.**

formatting: A process that prepares a *disk* to record data by creating tracks (like record grooves) and sectors (like pie slices) in its magnetic media. The combination of tracks and sectors act as a map into which the data will be etched. Most operating systems will prompt the user to launch an automatic disk formatting program whenever an unformatted disk is inserted into a drive. The term "format" may also refer to a prescribed arrangement of lines, margins, characters, and appearance that information entered by a user will automatically assume in a display.

fortuitous fix: A rare event in which a defect or bug in software is miraculously fixed while an unrelated part of the program is being worked on. The opposite phenomenon, described in *regression testing*, is much more common, wherein a single defect repair results in three new defects.

fragmentation: The necessary but undesirable splitting of data in a single *file* into fragments for storage in different places on a disk. This occurs because users add information to different files at different times, and disks operate on a no reservations basis in order to maximize the use of storage space. One still uses a complete file to work with, but, because the computer must gather the file components from noncontiguous places on the disk, the overall speed of operation is diminished. In defragmentation, a software program looks at the disk and shuffles data segments around to move data belonging to single files into contiguous blocks, similar to rearranging dominos.

function point analysis: A fascinating and very useful method of diagramming and estimating project application size. It breaks functional areas and features down into branching-related granular actions, sometimes to the level of single data field behavior, thus providing an excellent way to size the complexity and potential expense of development. A large project may contain 5,000-10,000 function points; an enormous one may contain 50,000 or more.

functional area (business area): Major business domains in an enterprise model. The highest level of compartmentalization is made up of subject areas, which are in turn made up of entities and their related data objects.

functional area owner (FAO): An individual responsible for a prescribed function or set of functions in a development project. The FAO is generally a *system analyst* with masochistic tendencies. The larger the project, the more FAOs required, because the number of design details that must be remembered by any one individual for documentation, testing, and implementation is enormous. **They do not really own anything.**

functional demonstration: The penultimate step in application development that occurs just before *roll-out* and after all designing, *coding*, and *testing*. It is the glorious time when *users*, *sponsors*, the project team, steering committees, and executives observe the full application, with all of its functionality, running in a special environment. **A marvel to behold, the functional demonstration is reminiscent of a graceful school of colorful angelfish, harmoniously darting in perfect unison with each other in a display of dazzling beauty. The code is then deployed to the dry land production environment.**

functional requirements: The critical initial components of any computer application development project gathered in *JAD* sessions and refined in *design documents*. They include descriptions of the precise inputs to the system, processes to be performed by the program, interactions of users with the computer, outputs of the program, and detailed information about the volumes of data to be handled, performance criteria, anticipated network traffic, hardware configurations, and user constraints on the system. Sometimes, technical elements of the functional requirements are delineated in a separate technical requirements document. **One should buy insurance against possible inaccuracy in these requirements and begin plans for spending the money.**

G

Gantt chart: An almost indecipherable geometric graph/chart hybrid that plots tasks in a project by subject area or individual against time. The resulting overlapping bar indicators are used to determine when resources should be added or subtracted, when critical pathways will be negotiated, and when team members are most likely to be calling the crisis hot line. Tasks that must be completed before others can be started are called critical dependencies and are supposed to be more obvious in a display such as this. **Some suspect that the hybridization reflects the genetic endowment of the banjo player on the porch in "Deliverance." Others think the chart amounts to nothing more than the waste of a "t".**

gap analysis: The evaluation and elucidation of the effort, expense, and time involved in moving from the present state to a desirable future state: Often part of cost/efficiency studies.

gland: Single-cell or multicell secretory units whose purpose is to produce and distribute substances of importance to an organism. Glands of the *endocrine system* secrete hormones into the fluid bathing them, which are picked up for distribution by the bloodstream to the cells they will influence from a distance.

goal: A specific defined target that a business has set out to achieve, ideally in support of the enterprise's overall mission. Goals should help to create strategic and tactical business plans. Information system projects should be aligned with the overall goals and mission of the business. Goals are distinguished from ideals because they are well understood and realistically attainable. **A goal might be to tell someone truthfully where you were when a meeting was held. Honesty would be the ideal.**

graceful degradation: A term used to describe a delicate way in which a program crashes, wherein users are warned of impending failure and functions are lost in a gradual and minimally disturbing way. The end result, graceful or clumsy, is the same.

Golbus' First Law: "No major computer system is ever installed on time, within budget, with the same staff that started it, nor does the project fully do what it's supposed to do."[7] Corollary to *Golbus' First Law*: Yours is unlikely to be the first.

graphical user interface (GUI): A style of screen interaction with a computer in which typed commands are replaced by manipulations of pictures *(icons)*, buttons, and menus via use of the mouse. This method is employed in windows types of operating systems, first popularized by Macintosh. It dominates the world of computing because of its intuitive ease of use, relieving users of the command line [C:*.*] typing that was required in the DOS world.

GUI: (see graphical user interface)

H

HTML (Hyper Text Markup Language): A standard way of displaying information that allows one to launch from a picture or word in one document to another document or web site that has been programmatically linked to it.

HTTP (Hyper Text Transport Protocol): The underlying communications protocol that enables use of hypertext linking.

hacker: A term describing a dedicated, somewhat obsessed computer aficionado (sometimes also called a "techie"), generally one who possesses superior knowledge in the area. Hacker has been unfairly used to describe someone who steals, defiles, or breaches the information systems of another. My preferred term for such criminals is *compoacher*. **Such individuals are often outcasts and subjects of fear and scorn, until those around them purchase a computer, after which they become the closest thing to a blood relation.**

hard-coded: A term meaning that the content of each screen that a user sees is the direct result of software instructions. Newer technology allows the content of the screens to be determined by choices that the user makes and controls through interactions with *knowledge* bases, and this means that the displays change without the necessity of code revisions.

hard-wired: Refers to the direct connection of one computer to another by cable dedicated to this purpose, as distinct from networks using modems and telecommunication lines. Like hard-coding, hard-wiring is a restrictive practice to be avoided when possible. **In fact, almost anything hard should be avoided.**

hardware: A term referring to the physical elements of an information system, other than users, that can be broken with a hammer. Basically, computers and peripheral devices.

help desk: A kind of system support within *user services* structured in a fashion that allows a very frustrated and angry user, in the midst of a tumultuous schedule, to call a convenient phone number that is reliably busy. **In the event that human contact is initiated, Mad's rule is invoked: The degree of help delivered is inversely proportional to the amount of agitation present in the user and always approximates the value of the help attained by a busy signal.**

---

high level: A term meaning general, vague, poorly defined, and not well understood, as opposed to *low level*, which means very detailed, specific, clearly defined, but still poorly understood. These interesting, but confusing terms are counterintuitive and therefore quite popular among managers. Not to be confused with a "high level of understanding"; the "of" makes all the difference.

homeostasis: From the Greek word meaning "standing the same," it refers to the state in living systems in which physical and chemical conditions and energy balance in the internal environment are stabilized with respect to surroundings and kept within a beneficial range.

hormone: Any of a number of messaging or signaling molecules secreted by glands of the *endocrine system* (and some nerves) that travel in the bloodstream and influence activities or events in target cells.

hot swap: The rapid exchange of a piece of malfunctioning equipment from a readily available stock of replacements by someone who knows what they are doing.

I

icon: A small picture on a computer screen that represents a program, a file, or an action that one can initiate by clicking on it with the mouse. Icons are the key elements of a graphical user interface that make it unnecessary for a user to remember commands, as was the case in days of yore. The icons usually look like the action one wishes to take (a printer, a shredder, an application logo). **They generally also carry a label for those who abhor icontact.**

identification: Who you are to a computer or network security system.

implementation: The combination of change management, infrastructure establishment, user education and training, application delivery, and information system support that constitute installation of an information system project in an enterprise.

informatics: Shortened form of the more illuminating "medical informatics," referring to theoretical and practical aspects of information management and communication in medicine and health care. It is derived from the French *informatique medical*; prior to 1975 it was called medical computer science, computers in medicine, health informatics, and a host of other arcane terms. **A specialty with this many names has a lot of nerve calling for a standard controlled terminology, n'cest pas?**

infobia: A term referring to the combination of fear of appearing incompetent while using new information system technology with fear of the effects of the information itself on job position, security, or personal adequacy. A very complex amalgam of human emotional responses to the perceived threats of new equipment and shifts in work processes driven by information-based assessments. The only word in this entire book that you have to know to pass the course.

information: A collection of facts or data with very specific characteristics—comprehensibility, relevance, availability, completeness, clarity, and comparability—in the possession of those who will use it.

information system architecture: The configuration, structure, and relationships of hardware (*computers, routers, bridges,* network connectors, *peripherals,* etc.) in an information system. Mainframe architecture is most familiar—a single *central processing unit* with multiple *dumb terminals* wired into it that users manipulate to enter and retrieve data. The terminals in this case have no brains, and therefore cannot be clients (although some have challenged this, pointing out clients who have no brains). This differs from *client-server* architecture where a larger computer (the server) is connected to other computers (clients), which may in turn be connected to even more computers (third-tier clients). A rule of thumb is that any computer that sends information to another computer is a server, and if it receives information from another computer it is a client. A computer can be a client and a server at the same time. This explanation is why very complex diagrams are needed to represent and illustrate system architecture. **Even system architects don't understand this stuff, but the language is very impressive at cocktail parties.**

information system: A system of hardware, software networks, and users, of which the last are the major component, that functions to collect, communicate, and evaluate data and transform them into information that supports the goals of an organization.

infrastructure: The underlying base of a system that enables its function. Often refers to the hardware and operating system software and network structure needed to enable complete information system function. It can also be used to refer to the foundation of business processes that enable *homeostasis* and healthy transitions.

Integrated Services Digital Network: (see ISDN)

integration: The incredibly complex and arduous task of ensuring that all the elements and platforms of an information system communicate and act as a uniform entity. This requires communication protocols, interfaces, cooperative human efforts, and standards. **And a miracle.**

integrator: In terms of homeostasis, one of three essential elements (the other two being sensors and effectors) that receive bits of information, process them, and initiate a response to the stimulus. **The brain is the ultimate integrator in most individuals.**

intellectual property: A term referring to creative thoughts, when such ideas are captured and documented before anyone else can prove that they thought of them first. When such thoughts can generate a solution, they may take on *value.* At that point, they become worth stealing and therefore worth protecting. **There are many laws referring to intellectual property, but a relatively simple way of determining if ideas may be valuable is to apply Samuel Johnson's sound judgment: "The work is both good and original; but the part that is good is not original, and the part that is original is not good.") This quote is attributed to Samuel Johnson, but it is not in the endnotes because neither I nor true scholars have been able to find such an aphorism in his works.**

interface: The zone between different computer systems across which complex messages are passed. Interfaces are the undeniable weak link of any system integration effort. There are emerging standards, common languages, and interface engines for the purpose of facilitating interfaces between systems. **One can observe a very impressive phenomenon with interface creations, reminiscent of the mating of the tiny male Australian Red Backed spider and its enormous female mate; even before full completion of the interface, the smaller of the two is being devoured.**

Internet: A rapidly growing world wide network of interconnected computers to which anyone with a modem and a service provider may attach and navigate. A portion of it is called the World Wide Web, which resource is revolutionizing mail, education, research, and business. It is low cost and enormously diverse, with connections to large databases and servers of all sizes across the globe. Graphical user interface browsing and searching software (Excite, Yahoo, Lycos, etc.) allow easy transmission of audio, graphic, video, and text files to anyone with a computer and a connection.

ISDN (Integrated Services Digital Network): A new type of network system that transmits voice, data, and signaling with complete *digital* end-to-end circuits and significantly increased *bandwidth* compared to traditional T-1 lines. Connection to this growing network requires an ISDN terminal adapter, which connects standard *modems* to the ISDN line. Ultimately, ISDN *digital* lines will replace current analog lines, at which time modems will no longer be necessary because their role in converting digital to analog and vice versa will be unnecessary.

issue: A euphemistic term for incomplete comprehension of an aspect of a project, applied when no one can ascertain if a PCR should be written, another JAD session convened, or more drastic personnel action undertaken to solve a new problem. **Also referred to as insurmountable opportunities, issues can multiply like bacteria. They represent the most common items in a project manager work session to be taken off line for resolution.**

iteration: The act of doing something repeatedly until one gets it right. Part of some kinds of project development methodology (rapid iterative prototyping), it cycles through design➠code➠test➠refine➠code➠test, ad nauseum.

J

JAD: A commonly used acronym for a Joint Application Design (or Development) session; a hyper-intense meeting of user and development experts in which requirements are detailed and system functionality is defined. **A properly executed JAD session results in extreme mental fatigue and irritability among participants and an all-important joint application design document. JADs are also referred to as Just Argued to Death or Jargon, Antagonism, and Diatribe sessions.**

Java: An object-oriented programming language related to C++ and used to create network-sharable, platform-independent applets.

K

knowledge base: A remarkable new way of representing data that transcends the common relational table *databases* so abundant in the systems of today. Information in a knowledge base is represented as individual concepts related to one another in a logical manner, through hierarchies of parents and children but also through meaningful links. A vastly superior way of representing large bodies of knowledge, such as medical terminology, it dwarfs the capabilities of current data storage methods because it has the ability to classify data concepts automatically on the basis of what the system knows about the concept, its definition, and its attributes. **A knowledge base almost thinks and, in this respect, is similar to a project executive.**

L

LAN: Acronym for local area network, referring to the technology that is required to support networked applications within a local environment (one department or building), not requiring phone lines for connection. **Distinction of LANs from WANs and other network configurations is unnecessary from a user perspective but important to maintenance and support personal who have to know on a moment-to-moment basis which station is down.**

laptop: A smaller than desktop personal computer that is more portable, but has amazing versatility.

learning curve: The period just after training in implementation when users are working with a new system in a production environment but are still learning and are therefore slower, less productive, and more stressed than normal. A critical period of installation when operational support is essential. **The only time a "flatline" is the preferred state of anything in the mind of the user.**

learning organization: An enterprise that is adept at gathering, disseminating, and using information to the benefit of the entire organization. It implies constant adjustment and change based on sensing internal conditions and external circumstances and facilitated through information systems and processes that best fit the business structure and culture.

logic module: A set of software rules or algorithms that instruct the computer to look at specific sets of data and draw conclusions based on them. The core of artificial intelligence.

log-on: The act of identifying oneself, passing security measures, and gaining access to a computer system or application.

low level: Low level means very detailed, specific, clearly defined.

Luddite: One who opposes technical or technological change; originating from the fictional Ned Ludd, leader of a band of saboteurs who destroyed mechanized weaving looms during the Industrial Revolution in England.

M

maintenance: Ongoing activities to support use and repair of an information system after deployment. This refers to fixing mutant bugs when they arise, updating code with enhancements, training and supporting new users, repairing equipment, monitoring networks, and tracking performance. **Maintenance costs are to the cost-benefit study as the iceberg was to the Titanic.**

MAN: Acronym for Metropolitan Area Network, a more ambitious network linkage over a wider geographic range requiring telephone lines within a city, versus more wide-ranging efforts often needing satellite communications (national/global). Most often referred to as its twin, the *WAN*.

management courage: The act of tactfully and diplomatically doing what is necessary to manage transition and deal with recalcitrant or antagonistic users. **As Al Capone is rumored to have said, "It is easier to get things done with a kind word and a gun than with a kind word alone."**

management discipline: Refers to the rigorous methods and intentions used to harvest the energy and the benefits from changes in business processes. The challenging act of actualizing energy gains from new processes that benefit the organization; the demand for tangible benefits as an energy carrier from processes in the enterprise that favor homeostasis.

management style: A term characterizing any of a set of behaviors or attitudes exhibited by a *project manager* in the course of performing his or her duties. Despite the fact that management style is almost always determined by the personality characteristics of the individual calling the shots, which couldn't be altered by much other than gene therapy, millions of dollars have been made by proponents of specific categories of demeanor. **Examples of these styles include principle-centered managers, tough-minded managers, managers with healthy habits, managers without spines, winning managers, sensitive managers of the nineties, Mafia managers, shark managers, and managers with similarities to Attilla the Hun, Prince Machiavelli, Al Capone, Cinderella, Boy George, and Chairman Mao. In reality, managers have ways of doing things that they apply indiscriminately, hoping to find an environment in which what they do works. To a leader who manages with a chain saw, everything looks like a tree.**

master person index (master patient index, MPI): A single unique person identifier used to reliably associate medical information with an individual. There can only be one MPI, which should be obvious from the descriptors "single" and "unique". **It's fun to test the sophistication**

of marketers who boast about their system's "MPI" by asking how they managed to obtain something that doesn't exist.

MCU: (see multipoint conferencing unit)

metabolic pathway: A series of steps within living organisms that facilitates the purposeful breakdown of substances or synthesis of materials needed to maintain homeostasis. These linear or cyclic processes are generally catalyzed by *enzymes* and controlled by *feedback loops* involving the products of pathways and influences from outside by relevant messages in a variety of forms.

metabolism: From the Greek word meaning "change," the total of physiochemical reactions by which living organisms acquire and utilize energy as they synthesize and break down materials in ways that promote homeostasis, growth, and reproduction.

microprocessor: (see CPU)

microprocessor controlled: Actions occurring under or initiated by an unknown, in a way nobody understands.

milestone: The term used initially in a project to indicate markers of progress, often tied to major deliverables. **By mid-project, these intervals will be replaced by footpebbles, and then by inchgrains as time goes on. This reflects the fact that the project team will simultaneously be dealing with a related entity, the millstone. Project managers have a millstone tethered to their necks at the beginning of the project for discipline and character building. They also use the millstone to demonstrate to their team the material they will be grinding their nose on as work proceeds.**

MIME: (multipurpose Internet mail extensions): A standard developed for transmission of nontextual information via e-mail. MIME attachments must be decoded by user e-mail programs through an SMTP (simple mail transfer protocol) gateway.

mission: The supreme overarching goal of an enterprise, usually described in a brief "mission statement." **The most impressive of these statements are developed by executives at off-site team buildings, generally congealing late at night after arduous discussion and sumptuous dining; these are called nocturnal missions. One wonders why some enterprises don't finish this important process, and why still others even begin it.**

modem: An acronym for the **m**odulator-**dem**odulator device that converts digital computer information into analog form so that it can be transmitted over regular phone lines to other computers. A variant is the Fax-modem, which allows the computer to receive data from a facsimile machine and to send data in a format that can be received by a fax machine. These useful *peripherals*, judged by their transmission speed, (measured in *bauds*), can be inside the computer casing (internal) or outside the casing (external) and plugged into a communication (COM) port. **Either way, modems emit a characteristic universal squealing, static, fingernails-on-a-chalk-board sound that managers should recognize as an indication that the user is about to cease all work-related tasks. Sophisticated users will want to obtain modem silencers, which are available at most gun and ammo shops.**

module: A logically related set of software code statements that can be connected to and nested within other instruction sets to build programs.

monitor: The peripheral device that contains the screen and the electronics necessary to present a visual display of programs and data for the user. Monitors come in monochrome (two colors only, one for image and one for background), grayscale (shades of gray), and color varieties. Some displays, called flat-panel screens, are not really monitors, because they use liquid crystals rather than traditional cathode rays to create the image (called LCDs—liquid crystal displays). Video cards control the monitors from within the computer and can determine the number of colors available and resolution of the image on the screen. Ratings of VGA (video graphics array), superVGA, and XGA indicate the general crispness, size, and color depth of the image on the monitor. **Anything with the word super in it is good.**

mosoneism: Extreme hatred of change or of anything new.[8]

motherboard: The fiberglass card to which the micro-electronics of the *central processing unit* are attached. Also called the "logic board."

mouse: A *peripheral device* shaped like the rodent and connected to the computer by its long tail. The mouse has a single ball in its underbelly and two or three buttons on its back. Moving the mouse to and fro on a foam device called a "mouse pad" circulates the ball, which, in turn, causes a pointer on the computer screen to move in the same direction. The mouse is useful only with a *graphical user interface (GUI)*, because its function is to help the user position the pointer over an icon, at which time depressing the left or right or both mouse buttons launches the program or actions signified by the picture. Not only can the buttons be depressed (called "clicking") once to cause an action, they can be clicked twice rapidly ("double clicking") to cause an entirely different screen behavior. Some mice have evolved a ball on their back, called a "track ball," that allows users to actually roll it directly with their fingers to control the pointer, rather than having to move the entire mouse around on its pad. Lately a new species of mouse has been observed, without a tail, that functions like the remote control of a television set. Electronic pen-pad and pressure-sensitive devices are also available that perform mouse-like functions.

moves, adds, and changes (MAC): Refers to addition, replacement, or removal of software features; moves or relocation of hardware; or changes or upgrades in modems, networks, or running software in an installed information system.

MPI: (see master person index)

multipoint conferencing unit (MCU): A special kind of bridge device that allows transmission of voice and video between networks. **The technology that has made the horrors of video conferencing a reality.**

multi-tasking: The capability of running two or more programs simultaneously on the same computer, with each program continuing to actively process data or perform tasks, regardless of which program is being viewed by the user. Multi-tasking requires something called "multithreading," which allows the *CPU* to diverge itself in a narrow wood, following both roads at the same time.

N

NC: (see network computer)

natural language processing: The process that occurs when a computer reads keyboard-entered text strings, separates the words or phrases into little packets (parsing), and assigns computer codes to the individual packets, thereby codifying the text for storage, analysis, and retrieval. One of the computer's most critical functions is to store and manipulate data entered by users, but it can only do so if the information is coded in a form that the computer can recognize. The language humans enter by typing or dictating is not coded and is referred to as "free text," and the words and concepts in the text have no meaning to the machine. If one has associated software codes with the words ahead of time, however, and if the user chooses these words from a drop-down menu or from a list on the screen, the computer knows what to do with them and can exercise its computational power on them.

network computer: Another name for a "thin client," a node with a CPU but no significant storage that is used to run programs on servers over a network rather than from programs stored on a hard drive.

network operating software (NOS): Programming that does for networks what *operating system software* does for computers. Nobody cares as long as the network is up. In the coding of medical terminology, for those of you who care, NOS means "not otherwise specified." People are working around the clock to eliminate this designation.

network topology: A term referring to the relationships of nodes and links in a network, often diagrammed when describing information system architecture. If you want a real treat, try to figure out how the term "topology" got thrown into the mix. It is relevant to anatomy (referring to physical relationships of organs or anatomic regions to each other) and to geometric theory (referring to properties of geometric objects that are invariant under continuous transformations), but otherwise was a term just waiting for some engineer to introduce into common misuse.

network: A system of computers and peripheral devices that are linked by communications media.

neural network: A complex web of interrelated nodes in an information system *network* that influence one another much as do the interlinked neurons in a nervous system.

neurotransmitter: One of a number of molecular substances released by nerve cells in response to a nerve impulse that act by stimulating receptors on the cell membranes of the tissues adjacent to the secreting nerve ending. Neurotransmitters are one class of chemical signaling molecules in living organisms that display characteristics completely analogous to those of *information* in a business setting.

NOS: (see network operating software)

nucleus: The part of a living cell that contains the hereditary endowment (DNA) and that is responsible for modulating many of the metabolic processes that occur within the cell *cytoplasm.*

O

object data model (ODM): Bundles of data and behavior grouped together in object-oriented programming.

object-oriented: Refers to a new way of programming and representing data using commands that act like little functional self-contained instruction or information units. These can be assembled or jumbled, aggregated or disaggregated, essentially treated like objects rather than like bits of data.

occupational community: A subculture group within an organization with common language, constructs of thought, background, and a sense of mutual identity. A lot like an organ or a tissue.

ODBC (open database connectivity): Standard specifications for connectivity between different systems in a Microsoft environment.

OLE (object linking and embedding): Object linking and embedding, an object programming technology for handling object components from varying platforms over a network.

open architecture: The state in which technical specifications for the design, structure, and operation of a complete computer system are revealed so that others can improve, modify, alter, create *peripherals* for, or *clone* the base unit. A noble ideal, sometimes combined with the concepts of *standards* and cross *platform* entities to convince the public that someday proprietary interests will vanish.

open system intercommunication (OSI): A standard conceptual communication model for establishing interoperability between networked systems. OSI defines seven layers. Physical (bottom layer): establishes the mechanical and electrical (cable) components and bit transmission. Data link: defines formatting of messages, synchronization, and encryption to be sent over the physical link. Network: defines routing, addressing, packaging (packet switching). Transport: provides end-to-end transmission control, error handling, resource optimization. Session: initiates the communication session, selects network services, deals with security and authentication. Presentation: provides format, code conversion, and data preparation for the interface so that users can understand the message. Application (top layer): provides end user interface services and defines how the user accesses the network. **May be thought of as analogous to the seven deadly sins, with "greed" at the application layer, progressing downward through lust, sloth, gluttony, covetousness, pride, and anger.**

operating system: The software that controls basic computer functions, such as preparing the file storage mechanisms, driving peripheral devices, managing memory, and interacting with applications. Examples are the disk operating system (DOS), UNIX, Windows, Macintosh-OS, OS-2, etc. The operating system, in combination with its hardware, constitutes a platform.

organelle: Any of several compartments of activities within the *cytoplasm* of the cell that are generally responsible for different metabolic pathways, allowing the metabolic processes to occur in a sequential and organized fashion. These include such things as mitochondria (which are key in capturing and using *ATP*), ribosomes (which manufacture proteins), and the *nucleus*.

organization matrix: Organization chart that maps roles and responsibilities rather than just indicates who gets to tell whom what to do. The chart displays those who are responsible for vertical project functions as well as those who are in charge of horizontal (cross-functional) areas. For example, one individual may be responsible for the order-entry and results-reporting function (vertical), but another is responsible for human factors and screen design across all functions (horizontal); hence a matrix. **This method eliminates hierarchical reporting of relationships and accurately conveys the fact that no one is really in control of anything, even though they are held responsible.**

OS/2: Operating System 2, developed by IBM with advanced capabilities over other operating systems at the time, the most significant of which was the capacity for multi-tasking. Now in a WARP version, soon to be Merlin, then....

OSI: (see open system intercommunication)

outsourcing: The act of going outside an enterprise for expertise in managing or maintaining a system, information or otherwise. This generally occurs when internal resources are inadequate, incompetent, uncooperative, or overly expensive.

P

Pareto Paradox: An often overlooked but extraordinarily important corollary to the famous Pareto Principle. The Pareto Principle states that "the significant items in a given group normally constitute a relatively small portion of the total items in the group. A majority of the items in the total will, even in the aggregate, be of relatively minor importance." Also known as the 80/20 law, it can be paraphrased by saying that, if a 100 percent effort is needed to develop all functionality for a set of users, 20 percent of the effort would yield functionality that would satisfy 80 percent of the users, and therefore 80 percent of the effort aggregate will be spent developing the code functions to satisfy the last 20 percent of users. Another twisted application of the principle is that every user will be 80 percent satisfied with the application because they will only find it inadequate 20 percent of the time. **This might lead one to cut a few corners, because, after all, if you satisfy 80 percent of the users all the time or all of the users 80 percent of the time, that is pretty good. The "Pareto Paradox" observes: There will be a small group of users who require the subset of functions omitted because of misinterpretation of the Pareto Principle 100 percent of the time in order to perform their job. This group will consist of articulate, influential, thought leaders who used to feel that automation was the right thing to do.**

password: Secret character sequences that are entered via keyboard and either assigned to or created by users. They are used to match against an official security database table in an information system to verify that the identified individual is entitled to gain access. A security screen is usually presented prompting the user to enter his or her official identification and then a password, after verification of which the *desk-top* is loaded.

PC: (see personal computer)

PCMCIA (personal computer memory card/international association): A standard computer input/output socket that will receive a special credit card sized computer board. These can be plugged into the computer to increase memory, provide fax/modem capacity, or to provide network connectivity. **Another critical term, along with "RAM" and "gigs of storage," used to impress others.**

PDA: (see personal digital assistant)

PDP: (see predelivery preparation)

performance: A term describing how quickly a system will execute its intended functions.

peripheral device: Any hardware device attached to a computer system with a function other than basic. *Printers*, CD-ROM drives, sound cards, and mice are examples of peripherals. To control and operate these peripherals, a computer must have software called "device drivers." New peripherals usually come with a disk containing the relevant drivers to be installed on the hard drive; in the newest systems, multiple device drivers are resident even before the peripheral is added. These newer computers are said to have "plug and play capability." **Users refer to this capability as "plug and pray."**

personal computer (PC): A computer specifically designed for personal use, wherein the owner can set *defaults* and preferences and control applications. It is a term that refers specifically to IBM and IBM *clone* computer systems and not to Apple-Macintosh systems, which function almost identically but are on a different platform.

personal computer memory card/international association: (see PCMCIA)

personal digital assistant (PDA): Computers smaller than *lap-tops* and notebooks with somewhat more limited capabilities, generally used for personal schedule management. Some can produce a mean spreadsheet and load a vicious game of Tetris.

phase: A group of tasks, swizzled with steps and activities that, when performed in concert, result in a major set of deliverables. Different from a "stage,"although it's unknown how. **Work's generally organized in phases when contained delays, rather than abject failure, are anticipated.**

pilot: A vague term referring to the first introduction of new software into a production atmosphere. Pilot users are afforded the opportunity to use the program to be sure that there are no problems with the code,and to demonstrate application usefulness in the trenches. **Putting code into pilot is very much like sticking one's toe into the water before plunging in. A successful pilot ensures temperate conditions for roll-out and confers the confidence needed for the project team to execute its graceful dive into the shallow end of the pool.**

PING (Packet Internet Groper): The act of sending a manual or an automatic message (echo request) from one computer to another over

TCP/IP network to ensure that the recipient is ready to receive messages and perform intended functions. **This allows system administrators to assure users that the system is up as they stare at an error message on their workstations that states that the system's down.**

pipe: A communication pathway established between servers or other networked computers. Inability to establish a pipe leads to a pipe error. **Exactly how a pipe is different from any other kind of connection that allow computers to communicate is uncertain, but it certainly sounds better when used in combination with the term ping.**

platform: A term referring to the combination of hardware and operating system software that an application can run on. A *personal computer* with OS-2 is a platform that can run IBM compatible software; the same software will not be compatible with an Apple computer Macintosh operating system platform. Some software can be run on multiple platforms (and is therefore called a "cross-platform" application). Other programs must be converted, or "ported," onto different platforms in order to be executable.

POP (post office protocol): A mechanism that allows servers to store mail for users until they are ready to access.

positive feedback loop: Operation in which the products of a transition or transition process cause the process to be speeded up or augmented. Organisms sense conditions and use feedback loops to regulate activities. In business, the most effective such loop is the positive thinking feedback loop, which is invoked when users recognize the benefits of an induced change and think creatively about additional methods for improving performance as a result.

predelivery preparation (PDP): Getting physical sites ready for the new system, including such things as placing purchase or lease orders; receiving; unpacking; assembling; configuring; testing; and, in some cases, repackaging and moving systems to the work site. Transportation and storage of the equipment, on-site set-up, and asset management also are elements of site preparation.

printer: A hardware *peripheral* device that converts files into printed paper pages. Printers come in numerous varieties, of which dot matrix, laser, ink-jet, and thermal transfer are examples.

problem: Anything that hinders or prevents the achievement of a stated goal. Sometimes referred to as an opportunity by inexperienced morons. **Those who have achieved true wisdom know that careful analysis of a problem serves only to increase its complexity. If everyone threw all their problems into one pile, they would kill each other to recover their own "opportunities."**

programming language: Also called "coding language," it refers to word and symbol sequences that are understandable to humans and that can be *compiled* into binary messages (bits) that are understandable by computer processors. The language that the humans use is called "high-level" language, and, to a certain degree, it resembles natural human language (nonprogrammers can make out a word or two). There are two major families of high-level programming language. The procedural family relies on an information frame (think skeleton) and a set of procedures (think muscles) that work together to make purposeful motion (examples are Pascal, C, FORTRAN, COBOL, and BASIC). The object-oriented family uses functional units (think entire individual joint with bones and muscles) that can be assembled in different ways (examples are C++, SmallTalk, Java, and FORTH). Regardless of which family of high-level language is used, another program (a *compiler*) will be needed to translate the instructions into more atomic codes that can be understood by individual processors; this translation process generates "low-level language," also called "machine code," which is directly responsible for computer board actions. **Really low-level language is employed by comedians, adolescents, and a few remaining longshoremen.**

progress: An elusive mystical phenomenon in large projects that some experts in the field believe does not really exist. **Others believe that progress is real, and even good in a project, but that it generally tends to go on too long. Remember the admonition that, given sufficient time, nothing can be done.**

project: A series of activities performed to obtain a goal. The activities are described in a project plan and are assigned to project team members by a *project manager*.

project change request (PCR): The most critical element of any fixed price or limited scope project, the PCR is a formal mechanism used by partners (or opponents) to present each other with items they believe they should either obtain for free or provide at exorbitant cost during project development. PCRs may be generated by any project participants and given to managers, thereby documenting design concerns or delivery problems requiring attention. **PCRs may generate additional costs or time delays, but they always serve to distract managers from real work. There are nuances to PCRs (investigation versus implementation, issues versus defects, what was said versus what was written down, etc.) that must be mastered by project managers before they can ascend to the ranks of project executives.**

project executive: A supreme manager who has ascended from the ranks of project managers by virtue of dedication, brilliance, wisdom, and indomitable spirit. Individuals in this position are experienced and specially certified in conflict management. **Project executives are important because they will lose their jobs if their projects are not successful. How this differs from the remainder of individuals on project who will also lose their jobs if the projects are not successful is a great mystery in upper-level management.**

project manager: A person or persons responsible for controlling project scope and for guiding efforts in obtaining the goals and directives set forth in the *statement of work*. **These leaders require very specific skills: the ability to argue an unarguable point of view; blind spots ensuring proper internal and external design documents; mild manic-depressive disorder with axis 2 anxiety characteristics; congenital absence of the compromise center in the cortico-medullary tracts of the midbrain; the specific, and rare, ability to spontaneously suggest untenable solutions to problems others more qualified than they have spent months analyzing. Project managers are optimists, the**

basis of which is sheer terror. They are ultimately responsible for failures, whereas the *steering committee* is relied on to shoulder successes.

project manager work session: A very important scheduled time for managers to meet and address cost overruns; schedule delays; issues; user concerns; *steering committee* concerns; PCRs; and, if there is time, successes. **The most fruitful of these meetings involve updating of resumes.**

project plan: A complex, time-oriented display of elements of a project with critical interrelationships and overlapping critical pathways. Using tools such as *function point analysis* and Gantt charts, it produces graphical representations of the plan that rival the complexity of the engineering diagrams for the boring electron microscope. **These plans are critical for determining the inadequacy of resources for the scope of work and for quantifying expected time and cost overruns (Golbus 1st Law).**

project review: A process of critical review of a project by a set of impartial observers for the ostensible purpose of suggesting changes to improve *progress* and maximize chances of success. Project reviewers are masters of observation and tact and are skilled in discovering how things are really going from all involved parties. **Immature project managers may be intimidated by project reviewers, but mature managers understand the diplomatically delivered criticism of reviewers: "We enjoyed your internal and external design documents; who wrote them for you?" To which the seasoned manager responds: "I'm so glad you liked them; who read them to you?"**

project sponsor: The key visionary responsible for the genesis of a project. Typically in charge of the *cost-benefit* analysis and the tactical maneuvers to sell the vision to upper-level management, he or she also shoulders responsibility for putting together the project team and providing direction to get things rolling. In the area of information systems, the sponsor is often also the chief information officer (CIO) of the organization. **CIO is also an initialism for "career is over."**

project status: A word referring to a confusing, volatile, graphical display of project tasks started versus project tasks expected to have started or of tasks expected to be completed versus those actually completed. Project status reports are, of course, required by the steering committee. **Even when a task is actually completed, members of the steering committee can be expected to express sentiments identical to those of a pallbearer at Houdini's funeral, who is rumored to have said, "Bet you a grand he isn't in there." Because this is a tool to specifically document and follow project progress, it may be viewed as unnecessary.**

project vision: The initial, very important element of a project that describes the goals and reasons for embarking on the work in the first place. This solidly grounded foundation and set of principles will be visited repeatedly during design and implementation to provide solace for enduring the excruciating tribulations of system development. It must clearly align with business plans and expectations and must soothe those who will be funding the effort. **As Edward R. Murrow observed, "The obscure we see eventually, the completely apparent takes longer."**[9]

protein: A type of molecule made up of one or more chains of building block molecules called amino acids. The order of these amino acid chains (also called polypeptides) is determined by messengers from the cell nucleus, is based on DNA gene sequences, and causes the large molecules to fold up in a specific three-dimensional manner. This folding is what configures the molecules for action if they are enzymes and gives them meaningful shape if they are to be signaling or receptor entities.

protein receptor: A kind of protein that generally resides as an embedded element of the cell membrane and that has a binding site that can be activated by chemicals or other messaging molecules. When appropriately signaled, these proteins can induce regulatory changes in the membrane or signal the cytoplasm organelles or nucleus of the event.

protocol: A term referring to a specific set of rules governing the manner in which information is exchanged over a communications network. Sometimes confused with algorithms, which are similar rule sets but are not generally applied to networks. Protocols define formats and sequences of messages and set forth methods for error handling, independent of the network hardware or communication medium.

prototype: From the Greek word "prot," meaning first, or primitive. This term in software lingo refers to a set of computer screens meant to illustrate what a user might see in the end product, conveying the idea that the observed manipulations will ultimately cause something to happen. This prototype is fantasy-ware, without architecture, communications, data, or infrastructure to support it. **A term identical to the above, but referring to a product marketed to unsuspecting buyers by competitors. Also called a demo. It is also sometimes used to refer to the first incarnation of a full-fledged system, delivered in a futile attempt to meet a delivery date, or milestone, possessing an astronomically high expectation of failure.**

protozoan: Single-celled living organism with a nucleus, *cytoplasm*, and *cell membrane* that serves as a model of relatively solitary operation in the bio-enterprise framework. Protozoans were initially named "first animals" and have classes based on their methods of motility (ameboid pseudopods, flagella, cilia) or on their ability to form infectious spores at some point in their lifecycles.

Q

Quack: A pretender to medical skills, a fake practitioner. Practitioners who continue to please their customers but not their colleagues.[10]

R

RAM: (see random access memory)
random access memory (RAM): The boards that handle information and programs in *real time* on a computer as the user manipulates the screens, selecting information from the much larger hard drive and mak-

ing it instantly available for use. This information is ephemeral (not stored) and therefore will vanish forever if the computer is powered off during a work session. It is important to save information to the hard disk frequently while working so that it is not lost when the dog steps on the power strip on-off switch. If you like to *multi-task* (do several things at once) or to have several programs running at the same time, you will need at least 16 megabytes of RAM. Second only to the size of the hard drive in impressing others with your hardware is the amount of RAM you have on a system. **You will also need to master the fine art of communicating this fact with panache: "I have a 2 gig drive, 32 meg o'ram, 200 hertz of screaming power, dude." Try to do this repeatedly immediately after you get your system, but only for a couple of months; then act smug in your confidence by being strongly silent. In actuality, the likelihood is that your system was obsolete when you bought it, and the next person you attempt to impress will skewer you like a pithed frog.**

rapid iterative prototyping: Describes a unique example of a core *development methodology* in that any combination of two of its terms is an oxymoron. **There is no English expression I am aware of that describes the situation represented here, in which three incompatible terms are placed together to represent a single concept.**

reactant: A substance that is acted on in a transition and changed to an end product, also called a substrate.

real-time processing: A kind of ongoing computer processing in which any change on the system is immediately recorded, files are updated, and displays are refreshed as they happen, thus approximating real-world operations. This is in distinction to batch processing, in which actions are stored and processed later, all at one time. **Occasionally, real-time and batch processing can coexist, as with some appointment systems in which appointments are booked and displayed to appointment makers in real time but are downloaded to users in a single batch process at night, when they aren't there to see them.**

recursion: A term of mathematical relevance from the Latin, *recurrere*, which means to run back. In math, it means that each number of a polynomial expression is determined by the recursive application of a formula to the preceding number. In information systems, it applies to programs that call on themselves to complete a task they have begun. **In management, the act of calling on oneself to complete a task—i.e., leaving a voice mail reminder in one's own mailbox—is a unique form of recursion that should be lauded as a highly sophisticated formal mathematical practice and not as an embarrassment to the feebleminded imbeciles who employ the technique. Recursion also refers to the forceful and repetitive use of a single expletive when a computer system malfunctions.**

redundancy: A unique term in information systems that has a meaning autonomous to the one generally acknowledged in English language dictionaries. Whereas in everyday usage redundancy means superfluous and unnecessary, in the world of data it means essential and indispensable. Because there is virtually a 100 percent chance that any data element or program can be damaged or lost (called a *disaster*), information system architects apply preventive measures by redundantly duplicating each element or program and storing it for use in the event of a problem. **Sometimes called "mirroring," redundancy reaches a pinnacle in the form of disaster planning, in which all software code and data are duplicated and stored off site. This practice is enormously expensive, but it ensures that volcanic eruption or antediluvian flooding will not be the element responsible for bringing the organization to its knees.**

reengineering: The process of painfully reordering human activities for adaptation to the requirements of an automated system (which was developed with the explicit intention of *not* necessitating reengineering). **The champion of reengineering is often in the position of a prisoner, pilloried face up in the lunette of a guillotine, giving well-grounded instructions on how to correct the defect in the instrument that is preventing the blade from its expected descent.**

release: A delivery of software to testers or users in unfinished form, with a numeric designation that contains a decimal and several digits. Releases are sometimes called "versions." As a rule, a higher or more impressive version number (e.g., 5.235) indicates a less satisfactory development process. **Developers who finally succeed at delivering a release have been observed to jubilantly chant in unison: "We're number 1.2!"**

reliability: A term referring to the ability of a system to perform its functions without errors, crashes, or performance problems. Sometimes measured as the mean time between failures. **A vendor that claims an extremely high mean time between failures may also claim to be a fat anorexic.**

remote operations service element: (see ROSE)

replanning: The mandatory process of completely reevaluating a project periodically during development. Replanning is enormously draining, as it entails shuffling resources, recreating time lines, swapping managers, and infusing complexity. **Projects that are in critical trouble will only have one or two of these costly entities, whereas those that are less moribund can count on replanning every six to eight months. Very successful efforts may need to step this rate up even more if they are to remain behind schedule.**

replicated architecture/technology: The new method of multiplying the shortcomings of mainframe computing into a network of occasionally communicating, smaller, separate computers, each of which is intended to serve as a back-up for another in the event of a point failure. **This technology gives the impression that performance will be optimized and that takeover functions will be a distinct advantage to users, ignoring the fact that there may be thousands of nonbacked-up points of failure that have nothing to do with the computers.**

resistance: Deliberate or subconscious actions that interfere with introduction of new systems or with the institution of change. In the information systems area, resistance ranges from complete rejection of an effort to sabotage, equipment damage, absenteeism, and organized protest. Falsification of information, data tampering, and rumor mongering are also features. Resistance is a normal and expected part of any transition, and management of transition energy is the lever with which organizations can influence stability in their enterprises.

Responsibility/Reward Principle: Introducing responsibility for data entry along with the reward of rapid information availability maximizes chances of global behavior changes necessary for adoption of a new computer system. Presenting all of the rewards of a system first and subsequently requiring user effort to meet overall organization goals has a high likelihood of failure.

RFI (Request for Information): A formal document developed by an *enterprise* and distributed to a set of vendors as an instrument to gather information about marketplace offerings. This is an early investigation tool that seduces vendors into thinking that they might actually be able to compete for an organization's business. (It also gives the false impression that the organization knows what it wants.)

RFP (Request for Proposal): A formal document generated after the RFIs have been evaluated, setting forth the precise requirements and questions relating to a desired system or service. RFPs are sent to a subset of vendors who are given an opportunity to further specify their offerings, answer questions, and indicate bid prices for their products. The details of RFPs are strictly confidential to avoid troublesome bickering among the contestants. **Skilled managers will try to find appropriate ways of leveraging the vendors without violating the business code of ethics, unless of course there is a deadline.**

risk: The omnipresent element of every decision or endeavor that forebodes failure. Concern about risk allows one to avoid examining the consequences of success. Minimizing risk is an important aspect of management, particularly as it applies to implementation of systems. In the field, minimizing risk means delivering a system that keeps morale high, improves productivity, eliminates duplication of effort, improves access to needed information, betters job satisfaction, and facilitates communication. **Because such a system has never actually been observed in any operation, some have determined that the ultimate in risk reduction is to promise nothing, do nothing, and be nothing, quietly. This approach, however, may mean success in losing one's job.**

roll-out: The process of deploying a system to users, often in a rapid sequential fashion, after development and extensive testing. Roll-out follows training of users, site preparation, network testing, and a *functional demonstration* of the software applications in an integrated environment. **Roll-out always occurs at the worst possible time in the organization and is considered a success if users are in turmoil but the system does not break.**

ROSE (Remote Operations Service Element): A very important service element that allows cooperation between two interacting applications. ROSE, like an executive, facilitates cooperation between clients and servers but does not know how to carry out the actual applications.
Rose's acronym: BOFIB, meaning bigger or faster is better.
router: A programmable device that receives and sends information

from one system to another without really doing anything but routing the information where it is supposed to go. Most often identified as telecommunications equipment, these handy devices can incorporate security measures, such as *passwords* and *call-backs*, and can greatly facilitate use of *client-server* applications and *distributed architecture*. **They are an important point of failure in complicated information systems and should be immediately blamed for any network problems that are experienced.**

S

scanning: Refers to the process of feeding a written, marked, or drawn paper document (or sometimes photographs) into a machine that transforms the image into a digitally stored replica that can be viewed and manipulated on line. In the case of writing or drawing, what you see is generally what was imaged, and you can't do much other than view it. Marked scanning, like that employed when one took the SATs, takes markings in prescribed places and puts them into a database that information systems can then manipulate. **Scanning is also involved in the unpleasant situation in which an individual's head explodes during a JAD session, immortalized in a movie (Scanners) several years ago.**

scope: The rigidly delimited and carefully described functional contents of a project the parties agree to in the *Statement of Work*. Scope is the raison d'être for *project managers*, because without it anyone could design, develop, and deploy a system without fuss. **Scope must be vigilantly policed by project managers, because designers, developers, and users have no self-control; if left to their own devices, they would delay a project until it actually met its originally conceived intentions.**

scope creep: The insidious process of project expansion that adds complexity and cost to an effort; the most common reason for not meeting a *milestone* or *deliverable*. **Scope creep was initially referred to as entropy by physicists in the immutable Second Law of Thermodynamics, which states that disorder in a system can never decrease and will always increase toward infinite randomness.**

scrub: The process of cleaning up a mess that has been caused by running a helpful application that has mistakenly intermingled crucial data with garbage. Scrubs require considerably more energy and diligence than just dumping a mess. Sometimes scrubs are necessary even when there is no mess, because a system has rendered information that is supposed to be acted on in the system unavailable, causing frustrated users to take care of the activities manually.

sensory receptors: Organs or molecular structures that sense stimuli or conditions and transmit information about the stimuli to other parts of an organism.

service levels: Expectations as to response time and quality of help available when problems become evident in a system.

shareware: Software that is posted on computer servers for network users to download for personal use. Usually, the software has an expiration date on it, after which time it threatens to self-destruct. Some, in fact, do stop working on that date, in the hope that you liked the sample so much you will go out and purchase a licensed version of the product. Others can be used beyond the expiration date. **It is embarrassing, however, to be showing off your computer and have the shareware screen indicate you are on day 123 of your 30-day trial.**

SGML (Standard Generalized Mark-Up Language): A robust meta-language for creating mark-up languages such as HTML, allowing automatic links between documents or web sites.

simple animal: A model in the *bio-enterprise framework* that resides between the sponge and the complex animal models, distinguished from the former by the presence of nerve tissue and neural function and from the latter (for purposes of the model) by lack of hormones.

single point of contact (SPOC): The one point of contact for users who are encountering system difficulties that cannot be addressed by on-site support. It should be readily accessible to users regardless of the nature of the difficulty the user has encountered.

site preparation: The process of readying physical facilities for delivery of information system components, including establishing a platform configuration (hardware, software, networks) and assessing room space, power availability and location, lighting, heating, ventilation, air conditioning, fire protection, and physical security.

site visit: The process of visiting a vendor's installed system at a production site in order to assess its performance and appropriateness for implementation in the potential purchaser's environment. **Generally most useful in revealing falsehoods and lies in the RFP, getting to know the company sales and marketing representatives, trying out new expensive restaurants, and escaping the grind of day-to-day work.**

SMTP (simple mail transfer protocol): A standard set of communication conventions for sending mail over the Internet. SMTP is used to transmit the e-mail to server POP store & forward programs, from which mail is retrieved by user clients.

sniffer: Any of several devices often attached to ethernet or token ring networks to monitor processes on the network. They collect statistics on nodes, timing, errors, protocols, and packet size and detail traffic history and routing information. They can locate network faults, performance problems, protocol errors, and OSI physical layer problems. They can also issue alarms and print reports.

software: Coded electronic signals that instruct computer hardware to perform specific functions. There is operating system software (disk operating system (DOS), Microsoft Windows, UNIX Macintosh Operating System, IBM OS-2), which enables the fundamental but uninteresting functions of the computer, and application software, which allows one to perform futile activities in an area of interest. More precisely, software consists of *bytes* of data that are strung together in a delimited series of related statements called a "module." Modules exist in a sort of caste system, with the bottom of the chain represented by the primitive "stub" module. Above the stub are levels of more sophisticated, but nevertheless incomplete modules, up to the level of the esteemed transaction level, or "T-level" module, which is capable of totally processing a transaction. When the set of software modules reaches a mysterious threshold size, the operating system suddenly finds that it can actually do something with them, at which point they graduate to the status of "program." If it is a small program that does something cute, it is called an "applet"; if it is a larger program or set of programs that allow initiation and completion of a significant task, thereby meeting user needs, it attains the rank of *application.*

sound card: A micro-electronic processor board that can receive analog sound signals, sample and reduce them into a *digital* format *(bits/bytes)*, and store them as files. The same cards can reproduce the sounds as directed by the *files* and play them over speakers.

source code: Software code in its high-level *programming language* form. One should ensure that software purchases in a development effort include the source code as a *deliverable*, particularly if the enterprise intends to do its own system *maintenance.* **Source code is analogous to the verbal commands given to a vicious guard dog; it behooves one to know the actions that will result from "kill" versus "sit." Simply buying the dog is insufficient.**

specialization: The process of developing more limited or directed function, thereby relinquishing the need to be a generalist in the cellular world. Greater integration and cooperation generally allows more specialization and has been thought to indicate further evolution.

speech recognition: A developing and nearly usable technology that allows computers to record utterances and automatically translate them into written language in real time. In specific domains, where similar words and phrases are used repeatedly, speech recognition has been useful for some time. It generally requires training the computer to recognize voice phonetics, but thereafter it may be operator-independent. **In domains in which speech is varied and verbalizations are unique, such as a novel by Charles Dickens or James Joyce, or the screenplay for Dumb and Dumber, or a management memorandum, it has little utility right now.**

sponge: A model in the bio-enterprise framework that is between the single-celled protozoan and the simple animal models, characterized by multicellular cooperation enabled by local cellular messages, but not yet at a level to contain tissues and, in particular, nerve tissue or function.

SQL (Structured Query Language): A command language for storing or retrieving data from relational database tables such as SYBASE or Oracle. One writes an SQL query, for example, to investigate database elements based on specific user defined parameters.

standards: Methods, protocols, or terminology agreed on by an industry to allow proprietary systems to operate successfully with one another. Standards are analogous to the universal three-pronged electrical plug for operation of different appliances; whether one plugs in an iron, a microwave oven, or a hair dryer, the standard plug permits the user to be burned or electrocuted. Examples of standards are *TC-PIP* for communications, *SGML* for data display, HL-7 for medical data interfaces, **and TTC (The Ten Commandments) for human conduct.**

statement of work (SOW): The SOW is an exhaustive document detailing agreements between parties as to deliverables, costs, and methods as well as general timelines and milestones for payments; also referred to as a contract. This critical element of a large project must be excruciatingly solidified prior to beginning development in order to preserve sanity among involved entities. It may take months to years to adequately refine. **Used as the cornerstone in determining what is in scope or out of scope, this essential baseline agreement has a singular defining trait: It is vague and subject to multiple interpretations.**

steady state: Refers to conditions in which a new system has been delivered and implemented and users are past the *learning curve* and enjoying a stable changed environment. **A myth.**

steering committee: An interested group of powerful organizational icons whose purpose is to support and guide the efforts of individuals mired in the actual design, development, implementation, and management of a project. These committee members are essential to the project. They must possess highly sophisticated knowledge about their organization's financial status. **They must also be able to point out deficiencies where none exist, instill doubt into otherwise confident project participants, minimize successes, throw in red herrings, and disband immediately if any real threat to success becomes apparent. These individuals need not have any direct knowledge of the issues or vicissitudes of the project.**

strategic planning: The ongoing process by an enterprise of assessing *cost-benefit*, *cost-efficiency*, and *risk* to guide decisions about future business endeavors. This work should rely on evaluation of past projects as well as on visionary insight into developing trends and technology. **Sometimes undertaken by steering committees or task forces, planning efforts should be expressly embraced by executive management lest they not understand later the recommendation to "advance to the rear."**

subculture: A label for a collection of human behaviors within a department, division, or functional area that are linked to one another by common tools, language, and abstract thought. Also called an *occupational community*.

subject area: Elements of a "functional area" in the second layer of an enterprise model made up of entities and their related data objects.

substrate: A substance that is acted on in a transition and changed to an end product; also called a reactant.

SWAG: Initialism for silly wild ass guess. The most frequent method of problem-solving in large, complex, distributed computing environments. **A technique perfected among high-level management and consulting firms.**

system administrator (sys admin): Sometimes also called a system operator (sysop), meaning the individual responsible for running supporting, and backing up a program or system. **They are well known for utterances such as "what the hell," "that is soooo weird," and "What's that grating noise?"**

system analyst: A uniquely qualified individual with a gift for accurately evaluating the details of a computer or business system, all of which must be aligned for adequate functioning of the whole. Chief emphasis of these evaluators is on "exception" definition and planning— the art of detailing all conceivable minutiae that could possibly go wrong. **This detailing has the benefit of diverting attention from the enormous gaffes made by requirement definers. If on appropriate medications, analysts are exceptionally good at going up alleys to see if they are blind.**

system documentation: A description of system function and operation at the time of delivery. It is of sufficient complexity to completely confuse users, for whom the document is intended, but lacking in necessary depth to be useful to those responsible for maintaining it. **This arcane document is most important as a repository for blame when the system fails and cannot be resuscitated.**

system security: A term referring to the relative safety of a system or network from intrusion or invasion by unauthorized and unsavory elements. Hardware, software, information, and network operation must all be protected to ensure security. Threats to security are sometimes classified in unique ways: internal versus external with respect to a network, intentional versus accidental, active versus passive, and classes D (least secure) to A (very secure). An extremely important element of medical systems, in which protection of patient confidentiality and assurance of data validity are critical. System security must guard against potential viruses, worms, hackers, and sniffers that can reach barriers and steal or destroy data. **Managed with encryption, passwords, and other devices, security systems can successfully impede access to all users.**

system testing: An ill-defined process of insanely repetitive software manipulations intended to reveal bugs or defects in the code. Examples of defects revealed through the use of *test scripts* include anomalies such as system *crashes*, hosing, implosion, and lockup. (There are several varieties of system testing: Internal system testing, done privately by developers to see how many *bugs* and *defects* they expect to deliver. *Integration testing*, done by user experts who foolishly attempt to evaluate the function of the code as it relies on *interfaces* to other systems. *Regression testing*, the sometimes automated but always inadequate retesting of all of the code after a defect is fixed because of the likelihood that the repair generated new defects in the software. Also refers to the startling childlike behavior observed in pathetically regressed testers after a prolonged session of script repetition. User *acceptance testing (UAT)*, begun after the first three tests are solidly completed. UAT uses an unsuspecting group of users to see how the code performs under conditions approximating production. These users will spend 80 percent of their time learning to successfully negotiate *test scripts* and 20 percent of their time breaking the system by doing what they will really need to be doing in the work environment,

This area of testing can be expected to surface more *defects* than the number discovered by the combination of all three previous testing methods. *Pilot testing*, evaluation of code by actual users in a production environment. It reveals occasional bugs in the software, but, more crucially, it outlines major design and development overhauls deemed mandatory by the testers for widespread user acceptance. It is important to note in this regard that each group of pilot testers will demand reversal of changes implemented in response to the demands of the preceding pilot testers.

system usability: A term describing the degree to which a system meets the intended needs of the user community. A weak point in many projects, generally revealed with blinding clarity at *roll-out*, it represents the true measure of the success of an effort. **User comments, such as "This does as much for my day as Saddam Hussein does for peace," or "These screens look like a cross between a Picasso and an explosion at a meat packing plant," represent undesirable outcomes.**

T

T-1 line: A U.S. standard digital *communications medium* composed of twisted wires in pairs. The wires can transmit 1,544,000 bits of data per second *(baud)* and can accommodate up to 24 voice conversations at one time. *Routers* and *bridges* are used to connect T-1 lines to computers or LANs.

tangent: The most common element of important meetings, tangents are sudden digressions from the topic at hand to irrelevant but much more fascinating areas of discourse. The job of the meeting facilitator is to continually maintain participant focus on the critical issue, because only then can a proper decision be made to take it off-line for resolution.

task: A logical unit of work as defined from a singe individual's point of view. Tasks are done when they are judged to be complete by a superior. **Some consider delegation of a task to be tantamount to completion, but this is a very advanced management concept that is out of the realm of this book.**

task force: A group of people charged with transforming visions and high-level plans into strategic plans, while spawning cost-benefit studies and requesting information. **This is an ironic term, because it usually accomplishes few tasks and generates little to no force.**

TCP/IP: Initialism for transmission control protocol/Internet protocol, a set of rules that function as a standard for preparing and sending signals between computers over lines of various kinds. An example of a fairly successful *standard*.

technical support: After start-up sustenance of the hardware, software, and networks such that a system is available to users.

technocentric: A term meaning centered on technology or technological methods. Often used to imply a lack of attention to human peculiarities that are integral to use of technology.

technocentric utopianism: A term referring to the ideology that all that is needed for success of an enterprise is superior technology and technological methods. **Run like hell anytime you see the word "utopia."**

terminal emulation: A nondescript term with several meanings: the act of a PC functioning as a terminal extension of a mainframe system, a popular low-expense solution to the more appropriate method of creating a true interface. **The name for the curious phenomenon when an intelligent workstation suddenly acts like a dumb terminal because the PC seeks to emulate the terminal's behavior. Also, the last time a subordinate acts like a superior before being relieved of his or her duties altogether.**

test script: A prescribed series of steps directing manipulation of an application to see if it does what it is supposed to do vis-à-vis the design documents. Test script writers are very important, because they must be able to translate detailed user requirements into simple execution protocols that any uneducated tester can negotiate. **Once these scripts have been run successfully, project developers can be very confident that it will take at least 10 minutes for users to disclose enormous problems with the code.**

thin client: A computer with processing capability (CPU) but no persistent storage mechanism (disk memory); it relies on data and applications on the host it accesses to be able to perform. It is smarter than a dumb terminal, but more forgetful than a fat client. It is also less expensive than a PC.

thrash: frenetic, useless, repetitive code execution on a CPU or hard drive that paralyzes its ability to initiate useful computation or communication.

tissues: A group of cells and intercellular substances that function cooperatively to carry out specialized functions in animals.

token ring: A type of *LAN* in which an attached computer or peripheral device gets an electronic "token" that allows it to transmit its data using the entire bandwidth of the communication medium connecting the units. The ring refers to the fact that the LAN is a closed loop. Faster than *ethernet*, a token ring can handle 30,000 64-byte packets per second.

tool-based solution: A computer "term du jour" that refers to the provision of a system made up of one or more flexible tools that allow construction or modification of functions by users. This is in contrast to *hard-coded* solutions, which require developers to make system *code* alterations when changes are necessary. Some people get this confused with the term "componentized," heightening the illusion that an integrated information system can be disassembled and distributed in useful pieces to those who don't want the whole thing. **Tool-based solutions shift maintenance risks from the developers, who understand the system, to users, who don't. They also allow developers to sell pieces of the solution to those who don't yet realize they need the whole product.**

topology: A term referring to the relationships of nodes and links in a network, often diagrammed when describing information system architecture. If you want a real treat, try to figure out how the term "topology" got thrown into the mix. It is relevant to anatomy (referring to physical relationships of organs or anatomic regions to one another) and to geometric theory (referring to properties of geometric objects that are invariant under continuous transformations), but otherwise it was a term just waiting for some engineer to introduce it into common misuse.

training: The sum of the important activities specifically directed at teaching users how to use a new system in the work environment. It contains *education*, of course, but is distinct from it in that its goals are more directed and focused. Training should be designed to optimize both learning and system acceptance, and it must minimize disruptions of ongoing operations. The best methods involve *"just enough"* training rather than regimented standard curricula that may overwhelm some, bore others, and permit toxic infobia to pollute the attitudes of more confident, malleable, or well-adjusted trainees. Focused and tailored, the training speeds transition to use of the new technology, accelerates "positive feed-back loop" formation, and enhances the rate at which benefits of the system for the company can be realized. The timing of training most appropriate is usually called "just in time," meaning that users can go immediately from training to operational programs in the production environment.

transition state energy: The energy level that must be achieved in order for a transformation or a change to proceed to conclusion without further effort. Sometimes equated with *activation energy*.

transmission control protocol/Internet protocol: (see TCP/IP)

turnkey system: A computer system that is ready to be dropped into an organization and turned on. Turnkey systems should include all necessary hardware, software, documentation, and training materials. Turnkey-lite systems, which include only software and training materials, are referred to as shrink-wrapped products. Turnkey systems of all kinds do not consider the enterprise model, functional requirements, or specific organization needs, but rather rely on reengineering the business to fit the system. **If the business changes associated with the transition to the new system are of any magnitude at all, success with a turnkey system is about as likely as having a quiet insightful discussion with one's teenager.**

U

uninterrupted power supply (UPS): An emergency power source that can provide a limited amount of back-up power to a computer or to network equipment in the event of total power loss. The UPS takes power from standard lines and passes it on to the supported equipment through a battery and an inverter. The battery supplies power when the lines are down, but the primary power path is still through the battery when the lines are up. **They are a reliable source of failure.**

URL (Uniform Resource Locator): The infamous string of alphanumeric characters that indicate a precise Internet address, along with the-protocol to access it. **A real life example: http:www.amazon.com/exec/obdos/subqt/home.html.4691-2250084-222533. Simple enough.**

UNIX: It's not an acronym or initialism for anything; it's a trademark name for an operating system originally designed for mainframe computers that has been optimized for multiple simultaneous users and endowed with *multi-tasking* capability. It is a cross-platform type of *operating system* capable of running on different types of computers and was written in an open (nonproprietary), high-level *programming language* called "C." This is a very popular operating system for development projects, but it's not very useful on PCs because it lacks a graphical user interface and is relatively complicated to use.

user: A human who interacts with any element of a information system in an attempt to enter data into it, retrieve data from it, or play games on it. **Sometimes called "grayware," referring to the user's brain matter (which is really pinkish white). A term employed by developers as a synonym for idiot, referring to those individuals who pay and revere them for their efforts. The most common reason for software and system malfunctions (see user error).**

user error: The term applied to the situation in which an individual using a program performs the most intuitive and most logical application action and gets a completely unexpected result.

user services: A section of most information systems departments responsible for setting up, maintaining, and troubleshooting computers and their applications for users. The usual initial contact with user services is through the *help desk*, which functions like well-done medical triage, enabling patients to get better on their own. This process is also called "empowerment." **Significant problems make their way up to computer technicians, who try to diagnose the problems remotely for several hours prior to working directly on the problem computer. Individuals in this role must be skilled therapists who can soothe the savage user and at the same time explain some arcane licensing agreement that prohibits them from upgrading the system so that it functions properly.**

V

vendor: Anyone who wants to sell you something. Different from a partner, in that there is typically very little risk sharing by the vendor. **Derived from Greek term meaning spiteful, deceitful, heinous enemy on whom I am entirely dependent.**

video card: A micro-electronic processor board that determines important features of the display on the *monitor* or screen. It defines the color depth and number, the resolution, and the speed at which images can be sequentially displayed (allowing for movies). Sometimes combined with a video accelerator board, which makes the video card even more powerful and fantastic.

video conference: An annoying technologically advanced method of meeting without traveling in which *multipoint conferencing units* allow video images and voice communication to supplant direct interaction. **The unflattering video images and aggravating delayed sound transmission magnify all of the miserable aspects of a meeting while eliminating meaningful human contact. One step above the teleconference (telephone without video), video conferences are often meted out as punishment by an angry steering committee. They are of greatest utility for scheduling the next face-to-face gathering.**

virus: A software program designed to damage computer data and programs and, in some cases, to erase hard disks entirely. These programs are communicable and travel on floppy disks from computer to computer or along networks through modems. They have varying degrees of virulence and may remain latent and undetectable on a system until the time they are programmed to hatch. Antivirus programs work to both prevent and eradicate infection, but they must be updated periodically to keep up with newly emerging strains.

W

WAN (wide area network): Refers to network technology required to support networked applications over a geographic range requiring telephone lines (a city or a state) or needing satellite communications (national/global). **The distinction is unnecessary from a user perspective, but it is important to maintenance and support personal, who have to know on a moment-to-moment basis which station is down.**

work flow manager (WFM): A new tool in computer systems allowing users to modify sets of object pathways (in the form of templates), thereby redefining the flow of information in the system. An object is presented to the WFM, which in turn hands it from entity to entity in the template along a chain to the end site. As the pathway is traversed, spin-off actions occur that may invoke parallel paths. The object is ultimately presented for manipulation or storage to its destination. **The WFM can be thought of as a "conductor," the Toscanini of the process, that assures that many individual actions produce the music intended by the composer. Toscanini was famous for occasionally referring to his orchestra as "assassins."**

workaround: A series of unnatural steps in a previously smooth operation that users must take to compensate for vagaries of a new software application. Workarounds are preferable to actually making code perform as designed so that delivery schedules can be maintained.

workstation: A super PC intended for individual use but with a specific work purpose and generally with bigger or faster work components than those of a home PC.

world wide web (WWW): The name of a portion of the Internet that has exploded in popuarity for entertainment, education, and business, sometimes called the information highway.

worm: A kind of computer virus that propagated over the *Internet* in 1988, crippling infected computers by reproducing endlessly and usurping computer memory. The worm creator was a graduate student at Cornell University named Robert Morris, who claimed that a piece of software he wrote to determine the number of computers on the net contained a bug that caused it to run amok. The courts didn't believe him. **The worm was successfully eradicated, but it has been preserved on magnetic media (tape) for posterity.**

WWW: (see world wide web)

WYSIWYG: Initialism for "what you see is what you get," referring to the fact that what you have entered on the screen is exactly what you will see on paper.

Every other author may aspire to praise; the lexicographer can only hope to escape reproach.—Samuel Johnson, English philosopher and lexicographer, 1775.

References

1. Excellent source for several computer-related initialisms, acronyms, and abbreviations is available at http://access.disexnet~ikind/babel96b.html.

2. Excellent online Dictionary of Computing available at http://instantweb.com/foldoc/.

3. Buckley, W. In Winokur, J., *The Portable Curmudgeon*. New York, N.Y.: New American Library, 1987.

4. Tenner, E. *Why Things Bite Back*. New York, N.Y.: Knopf, 1996, p. 14.

5. Turner, E. In Jarmen, C. *The Guinness Book of Poisonous Quotes*. Chicago, Ill.: Contemporary Books, 1993.

6. Bell, A. "Next-Generation Compact Discs." *Scientific American* 275(1):42-6, July 1996.

7. Worthley, J., and DiSalvio, P. *Managing Computers in Health Care*, Second Edition. Chicago, Ill.: Health Administration Press, 1989.

8. Attendorf, A., and Attendorf, T. *ISMS: A Compendium of Concepts, Doctrines, Traits, and Beliefs.* Memphis, Tenn.: Mustang Publishing Co., 1993

9. Murrow, E. In Esar, E., *20,000 Quips and Quotes*. New York, N.Y.: Doubleday and Co., 1968.

10. Starr, P. *The Social Transformation of American Medicine*. New York, N.Y.: Harper Collins, 1982, p. 23 (attributed to Everett Hughes.)

A

ABEND, 85
activation energy, 151
Active X, 82,101
adverse reactions, 10,32
AI, 89
algorithm, 81,104,118
American Cancer Society, 50
American College of Obstetrics and Gynecology, 50
American College of Radiology, 50,53
American Medical Association, 5,25
American National Standard Code for Information Interchange, 84
analog data, 92
ancestors, 10
antibiotics, 31,32
antisepsis, 14
Anti-Vaccination League, 17
application support, 191
application, 83,86
appropriateness, 61
architecture, 75,95
archiving, 112
artificial intelligence, 89
ASCII, 84
assessment, 1,27
Auenbruegger, Leopold, 17
authentication, 103
autonomy, XI,36
availability, 112

B

bacteria, 14
bandwidth, 91,96,97
baseband, 92
baseline document, 179
Basic, 81
baud, 96
big bang, 190

billing codes, 42
bio-enterprise framework, 126
biometrics, 103
bio-transition framework, 150
bit, 73,107
bleeding, 18
blob, 111
board, 75
BOFIB, 74
bone marrow transplant, 54
boot, 84
bottlenecks, 176
breast cancer, 50,51
bridge, 97
broadband, 92
Broussais, Victor, 18
browser, 100
browsing program, 100
bug, 85,112,180,192
business transition, 155
byte, 74,107

C

C, 81
C++, 82,101
callback modem, 96
cancer, 34,35,50,51
card, 75
cardipulmonary resuscitation, 30,54
catalysts, 153
CBT, 188
CD, 78
CDR, 111
CD-ROM, 79
Celsius, 12
central data repository, 111
central processing unit, 73,95
certification, 25
change management, 153,185
change, 150
chest x-ray, 49
chief complaints, 3
child-bed fever, 15
Chinese medicine, 11
chronic disease, 21

D

data dictionary, 109
data elements, 107
data files, 83
data model, 109
data pollution, 43
data storage, 77
data structure, 107
data toxicity, 38,42
data validity, 107
data warehouse, 58,111
database, 84,110
DCOM, 82
death march, 178
debugging, 85
defaults, 87
defect, 85,180,181,192
degradation, 93
deliverable, 176
delivery, 190
design documents, 178
desktop, 87
developers, 81
development, 178
digital data, 92
digital versatile disk, 79
directory, 84
disaster recovery, 112
disintermediation, 164
disk, 78
disposition, 60
distributed component object model, 82
divine intervention, 14
doctor-patient relationship, 13,21,47
documentation, 178
DOS, 84
drugs, 31
dual system, 190
due diligence, 175
Duh's Principle, 176
dumb terminal, 95
DVD, 79

E

EDR, 179
education, 24,161
effectors, 136
Egyptian civilization, 10
Einstein, Albert, 150
E-line, 99
enabler, 163
encryption modem, 96
encryption, 92,104
end products, 152
End-Stage Renal Disease, 49
energy carriers, 152,164
energy state diagram, 151
enterprise model, 109
enterprise structure, 125
entity, 108
entrance ramp, 100
entropy, 150,207
enzyme, 153
ergonomics, 157,186
ESRD, 49
Ethernet, 99
examination standards, 50
executable, 83
external design report, 179
extranet, 95

F

family history, 10
FAO, 180
fault tolerance, 112
fax-modem, 96
FDDI, 99
feature, 86
feedback, 165
feedback loops, 138
fiber digital data interface, 99
fiberoptic cable, 92,99
file, 83,84
file transfer protocol, 100
financial stakeholders, 23
firewall, 102

Flambé virus, 86
flattening, 125
Flexner, 26
floppy disk, 78
folk remedies, 25
format, 78
FORTH, 82
FORTRAN, 81
fragmentation, 40,78
free text, 88
Friday the 13th virus, 86
FTP, 100
function, 86
functional area owner, 180
functional demonstration, 183
functional requirements, 186
function point analysis, 176

G

Galen, 12
Gantt chart, 118,176
gigabyte, 74
goal, 109,172
Golbus' Law, 178
Gordon, Richard, 13,14
graphical user interface, 87
growth and development, 20
GUI, 87

H

hacker, 102
Halvorson, George, 29,61
hand washing, 15
hard boot, 84
hard disk, 78
hardware, 73,95
hard-wiring, 93
Harvard University, 26
Harvey, William, 12
health care triangle, 201
health care expenditures, 28
health risks, 10

health statistics, 29
HEDIS, V
help desk, 78,114,162,192,193
hierarchy, 125
high-level coding language, 81,83
Hippocrates, 12,13,25,35
history of present illness, 4
holographic data storage, 79
homeostasis, 127,150, 207
homo habilis, 10
horizontal function, 126
hormones, 139
hospitals, 32, 33
hot spare, 192
hot swap, 192
HTML, 101
HTTP, 101
humanity, 207
Huxley, Aldous, 209
HyperText Markup Language, 101
HyperText Transport Protocol, 101

I

iatrogenic disease, 33
identification, 103
IDR, 179
Illich, Ivan, 4
imaging, 22
Imhotep, 11
implementation, 185
infant mortality, 29
infection, 14
infobia, 27,38,43,120,149,155
informaciation, 27,38,57
information highway, 100
information system, 113
information system architecture, 95
information system therapy, 60
information technology changes, 199
infrastructure, 173
inoculation, 16
integrated services digital network, 96
integrated system, 39
integrated user interface, 58
integration testing, 181

integration, 105,111,141
integrators, 136
Intel Corporation, 75
intellectual property, 182
intensive care units, 30
intermittent defect, 181
internal design report, 179
internal system testing, 181
Internet, 82,85,95,100
intranet, 95
irregulars, 25,26
ISDN, 96
iteration, 182

J

JAD, 175,178
James, Geoffrey, X
JAVA, 82,101
Jenner, Edward, 16
Johnson, Samuel, 18
joint application design, 175,178
just-in-time training, 42,189

K

Kennedy-Kassebaum Bill, 29
kilobyte, 74
knowledge base, 111
Koch, Robert, 14
Konner, Melvin, 61
Kovner, Anthony, 34

L

Laennec, René, 17,18
LAN, 93,99
laparoscopic cholecystectomy, 48
leadership, 189
learning curve, 162,189,192
learning organization, 117,149
leeches, 18

legacy system, 141
Lister, Joseph, 14
local area network, 93,99
log on, 103
logic modules, 89
Louis, Pierre-Charles-Alexandre, 15,18
low-level coding language, 83
Luddism, 122,162

M

MAC, 194
Macintosh, 84,87
mainframe, 95
maintenance, 112
malpractice, 23
mammography, 49
MAN, 95
management courage, 193
management discipline, 153
management engineers, 173
mark-up language, 101
mass screening, 54
master person index, 57
MCU, 97
medical education, 24,46,47,59
medical language, 41
medical record, 11,19,38
medical records and rationale, 10
medical statistics, 19
medical terminology, 41
Medicare End Stage Renal Disease Program, 49
medications, 9,31
megabyte, 74
megahertz, 75
Mendelsohn, Robert, 4,7,33
memory, 79
Merlin, 84
metabolism, 127
metropolitan area network, 95
milestone, 177
mission, 109,118
modem, 77,96
modularity, 144
modules, 83
mosoneism, 46,122

mouse, 77
multipoint conferencing unit, 97
multi-tasking, 87

N

Napolean, 17
narcissistic personality disorder, 35
National Institutes of Health, 50
natural language processing, 88
NCQA, V
neonatal intensive care, 30
network architecture, 95
network computers, 96
network monitor, 99
networks, 91
network topology, 93,187
neurotransmitters, 137
normative validity, 54
nosocomial disease, 33
NPD, 35

O

object components, 82
object data models, 82
objective findings, 1,27
object linking and imbedding, 82
object-oriented database, 84
object-oriented language, 82
ODMA, 82
OLE, 82
open architecture, 76,101
open systems interconnection, 97
operating system, 84
optical compact disk, 78
organization matrix, 126
organizational structure, 125
OS-2 Warp, 84
OS-2, 87
OSI, 97
Osler, William, 49
otitis media, 31
outcome analysis, 156

P

packet, 97
Paleolithic era, 10
paper record, 39
papyrus, 10
paradoxical data toxicity, 27,42
parallel system, 190
Pareto Paradox, 158
Pareto Principle, 157
partner, 173
Pascal, 81
password, 103
past medical history, 8
Pasteur, Louis, 14
pathway, 48,53,156
patient identification number, 57
patient-doctor relationship, 13,21,47
PC, 76
PCMCIA, 80
PCR, 179
PDP, 187
Peabody, Francis, 208
Pentium®, 75
percussion, 17
performance, 112,183
peripheral device, 77,84
personal computer, 76
Personal Computer Memory Card International Association, 80
personal digital assistant, 76
pharmaceuticals, 31
phase, 177
PHS, 47
physician strikes, 33
pilot, 183
pilot testing, 182
plan, 1,56,176
platform, 76,111
platform configuration, 187
Plotkin, David, 50,51,53
point failure, 112
positive feedback loop, 165
Post-Hippocratic Syndrome, 38,47,155
practice patterns, 55
predelivery preparation, 187
prenatal care, 29
preventive maintenance, 194
problem-based progress notes, 39

procedural language, 81
professional beneficence, 36,47
program files, 83
programmers, 81
programming language, 81,177
project change request, 179
project executive, 174
project manager, 174
project plan, 176
project review, 180
project sponsor, 172
project status reports, 178
project vision, 172
protocol, 97
prototype, 182
protozoa, 127
protozoan model, 128
psychosocial factors, 9
Ptah, 11
puerperal fever, 15
pyramid of health care, 201

Q

Quantitative methods, 21

R

RAM, 79
rapid iterative prototyping, 182
reactants, 152
redundancy, 112
reengineering, 149,164
regression testing, 181
regulars, 25,26
relational database, 84
relational table, 111
release, 176,191
reliability, 112
remote operations service element, 98
replanning, 176
replicated technology, 112
request for information, 173
request for proposal, 173

resistance, 13,151
responsibility-reward principle, 191
return on investment, 172
RFI, 173
RFP, 173
Rifkin, Jeremy, 23,207
risk, 178
Robin, Eugene, 54
roll-out, 185
ROSE, 98
Rose's acronym, 74
router, 97
rubber gloves, 14
Rush, Benjamin, 18

S

scanner, 77
scope, 175
scope creep, 179
screening, 50,54
searching software, 101
security, 102
selective amnesia, 47
Semmelweiss, Ignaz, 15
sensory receptors, 136
server, 75,95
SGML, 101
shaman, 10
shared decision making, 37
shareware, 86
shotgun testing, 22
simple animal, 127,134
single point of contact, 193
site preparation, 186
site visits, 173
smallpox, 16
SmallTalk, 82
smart building, 93
SOAP, 1,39
soft boot, 85
software, 81
source code, 83
SOW, 175
speech recognition, 87
Spencer, Herbert, 171

T

topology, 93,187
trainers, 189
training, 161,187
transition state energy, 151
transmission control protocol/Internet protocol, 98,100
turnkey, 165,173
twisted pair cable, 91

U

V

W